**DEDICATION**
This book is dedicated to
Eunice Ingham, Pioneer of Reflexology,
Dwight Byers, our Mentor,
and all of our guests who visited
"The Last Resort."

Breeding Publishing
P.O. Box 10205
St. Petersburg, Florida 33733-0205

# PREFACE

This is *not an instruction book*. It is merely our way of sharing with you the results we have personally experienced through Reflexology therapy. It is *not* our intent to put down any medical therapy or physician. We believe that many times our body has the natural ability to heal itself when stimulated to do so. We believe Reflexology therapy is one means to help the body to normalize. Even so, we would *never* discourage anyone from receiving conventional Western medical assistance.

Reflexology is a science that deals with the principle that there are reflex areas in the feet and hands which correspond to all of the glands, organs and other parts of the body. Reflexology is a unique method of using the thumb and fingers on these reflex areas. Reflexology relieves stress and tension, improves nerve and blood supply, and helps nature to normalize the body. When we are using this method we say that we are "working" certain reflexes. The authors of this book feel blessed to be able to help people by using this natural, non-harmful therapy modality and discipline.

We chose the title *"Success At The Last Resort"* because most clients that have come to our office for Reflexology Therapy have already tried all of the conventional mainstream medical help available to them and it has failed. So many times Reflexology is *"The Last Resort"*.

When we began writing this book, in which we believe all of those serious about Reflexology will be interested, we considered whether to include case histories or only to make this a reference book. We decided to combine our ideas in order to make this book as practical and interesting as possible and to use case histories of our clients. Permission has been received from them, however, fictitious names have been used in most cases. There are many, many wonderful stories that other Reflexologists can tell. These are just a few of our true stories with some references as to how Reflexology was successful. Our client records show that over one thousand eight-hundred people have been to our offices for Reflexology consultations in the fifteen years that we have been in practice.

# ABOUT THE AUTHORS

How the writer, Diane Breeding, became a Reflexologist:

My husband suffers from chronic back pain. In 1981 I read a book, *Stories the Feet Can Tell* by Eunice Ingham. I began applying some of her suggested Reflexology techniques to my husband's feet. To my amazement his pain lessened and steadily began to decrease.

Later that same year, I received a schedule of The Original Ingham Method Seminars on Reflexology. In January 1982, I took my first seminar which was conducted by Eunice Ingham's nephew, Dwight Byers. It was "mind boggling." So much to learn! My thumbs can't walk! My first joint of my index finger has to do what? Bend? Walk? Never! ! By the end of the seminar, I was sure I had two left hands.

I went home and studied and studied and practiced on anyone, anywhere. If we were invited to friends' homes for dinner or card playing, Paul, my husband, would warn me ahead of time, "I don't want to find you on the floor at the end of the evening again." He didn't mean "passed out" or inebriated. By that he meant working on peoples' feet. And, I usually did end up on the floor with someone's foot in my hands.

Exactly one year after attending my first seminar, I became certified through the International Institute of Reflexology and began my new profession, Reflexology Therapy.

In 1984, I was very pleased to be invited by Dwight and Nancy Byers to do Reflexology sessions at their offices in St. Petersburg, Florida. That is where I worked the feet of my first paraplegic, my first spina bifida case, and my first multiple sclerosis client. I'm grateful for the experience I gained while working with them.

How Paul Breeding became a Reflexologist:

My husband, Paul, does not enjoy writing, but he has allowed me to interview him for this book. Why did Paul want to do Reflexology treatments for a living? He said, "My wife has proven that Reflexology works by eliminating my back pain. However, I may still have pain if I do foolish things; such as improper lifting or strenuous labor. After one or two Reflexology treatments, the pain is gone. I also wanted to get even with my wife, Diane. If she can give me discomfort while working my feet, then I should be able to do the same to her. I was Certified through the International Institute of Reflexology in 1989. Diane and I prove Reflexology and its benefits to people every day. We enjoy helping people."

"The proof is in the pudding." We offer a money- back guarantee. We don't recommend this to others unless they are *very* experienced. Our ad in the yellow pages says, "If we can't help, we won't charge." When a new client calls for an appointment, we explain that we need the first session to determine whether we feel Reflexology could be helpful. If we feel it is possible, then we ask for a specific number of treatments to be scheduled close together. After the agreed upon sessions, *if* the client can *honestly* say, "Reflexology has not been helpful," we will refund the payment. In the five years that this has been in effect, we have given money back only three times. Not a bad record!

Paul continues,

"When I began working clients at the International Institute, they were *all* "freebies." I had a list of names and numbers I received while doing Reflexology at a health fair. We had a drawing for one free Reflexology session. I called as many people as possible. I filled in any open appointments available. This was the beginning. I had to prove Reflexology in order to build my own clientele. Two months later, Diane and I opened our own office."

Paul's philosophy is that a positive environment is needed in which to practice Reflexology. A clean, pleasant environment is necessary. Clients want a relaxed treatment room with no screaming children, mates, or barking dogs - this is ideal for the quiet relaxation they need. He said, "I wish we didn't need our answering machine because it distracts. Our offices are simple, decorated with soft colors, background music, and windows that show off our beautiful oak trees. I'm not saying that there is silence, because if any one reading this book knows Diane, you know there will be laughter and happiness. We have good rapport and conversation with our clients. The majority of them enjoy our vacations through our pictures and stories. We send them post cards, get-well cards, and sometimes even anniversary cards. We do care about them and we try to show them that we care. They mean a lot more to us than just a fee for service rendered."

Our business cards say a lot when they say, "Put your feet in our hands." You can possess all the knowledge of anatomy of a top-notch physician. But if you *can't* do Reflexology successfully that is, see results, then you have missed the mark. To achieve results, you must gain sensitivity through touch. We are not believers in gentle Reflexology at our offices. We want to use deep pressure, and be able to ease up when necessary. You must be willing to practice with dedication and not necessarily always receive monetary compensation.

# CONTENTS

# SUCCESS AT THE "LAST RESORT" WITH :

## I. STROKE

Definition: A stroke is a sudden and severe attack caused by a rupture or blockage of a blood vessel in the brain, resulting in loss of consciousness, paralysis or other symptoms depending on the extent of brain damage.

(1) Jeff. There are frustrating times with Reflexology. I remember Paul's first feeling of frustration with a client who was suffering from a stroke which affected the right side. The stroke had occurred five years earlier. Jeff was bed-ridden, and if wheeled, could sit in a recliner. His left calf was grossly discolored and he had a lot of edema. Paul worked Reflexology on him at his condominium three evenings a week. The results were amazing. First, everyone noticed his speech coming back, next his right hand was able to open and close. Paul was so excited, he felt certain this man would eventually be up and walking, maybe not dancing, but walking with the aid of a walker.

At the fourth Reflexology treatment, we noticed that the left calf area became bright red and matter was flaking and dropping off. The area was not feverish, nor did it have an odor, but was scarlet in color. Jeff's wife was very concerned and told Paul that she was going to take him to the doctor before any more treatments. Paul thought, "This is it. The medical doctor will probably nix all further Reflexology treatment." The doctor told Jeff that the flaking was a build up of lotion that had been applied and not washed off. The redness was new skin. The doctor told him that the leg had the best circulation that it had since before the stroke. "Keep up the Reflexology", were the doctor's words.

Paul was delighted and continued with the sessions. The home health caregivers began applying vitamin E oil instead of lotions. Jeff was progressing rapidly. He was able to speak in short sentences and stand on his own. Suddenly we received a phone call canceling all future appointments. There was no explaination and we couldn't understand why his wife would want his treatments stopped. We couldn't believe it! Paul was crushed. Jeff passed away several months later. *Success, **then frustration!***

(2) Virginia.    She was eighty years old when she began Reflexololgy treatments to help her circulation and to get some of the edema out of her legs.  We were seeing great improvement in her legs.  Many times when Virginia came for a treatment her caregiver would tell us, "She's not doing well today.  She's not quite 'with it.'  She can hardly speak or walk."  Each time this happened we noticed some small reddish spots on her great toe.  When we worked extensively on these areas we could actually see Virginia perk up and come out of the clouds.  By the end of her hour-long Reflexology session, the reddish spots were pale pink or sometimes gone.  Virginia was like a different person.  After her treatments it was her treat to take her caregiver out for breakfast.  Virginia's  doctors had told her she was having mini strokes, or TIA's (trans ischemic attacks).  Virginia's main concern was not ending up in a nursing home.  Any time she acted strangely or listless her caregiver would call and bring her in for an appointment or we would make a house call.  Each time there were spots on her great toe.  This continued for six years and Virginia continued to stay in her own home until her final stroke in the middle of the night. We know Reflexology was responsible for providing Virginia with a better quality of lifestyle than she would have had without the Reflexology treatments she received.

(3) Bruce. Bruce's wife talked with us when we were exhibiting for a health fair at a local mall. Her husband had suffered a stroke and his prescribed rehabilitation was completed. His speech was fine, but the circulation in his legs and feet was so poor that he could barely walk. We told her that if she could get him to come to us while we were at the mall, he could receive a free Reflexology treatment on his feet. Within the hour, she had Bruce in our chair. His feet hurt so badly that he couldn't wear shoes. He wore extra large slippers and had to have assistance in order to get to our booth. Bruce was already a believer in Reflexology. He told us that had worked on his own feet and that he had books and charts on Reflexology. Bruce came to our office for five treatments. He experienced great improvement in both legs and feet. He also noticed an increase in his energy level. The evening after his fifth treatment, he went to Bible study at his place of worship. The people could hardly believe the difference. Paul always says, "The proof is in the pudding". This particular *success* story generated more than twenty new clients for us.

(4) Jenny. Jenny had suffered a stroke, which made her entire right side weak. Her speech was affected but she was understandable. When she came to our office, she dragged her right foot and leg. After just two Reflexology treatments, she was able to lift her leg and place the foot down. The first stroke she had was more than six years prior to coming to our offices. She had experienced all of the therapy prescribed by the doctors and was left with her leg dragging as she attempted to walk. Reflexology not only helped her leg and foot but she realized an improvement in her speech as well.

When we performed Reflexology on clients who had suffered with strokes, we found the following reflexes to be the most helpful: *brain, (on the opposite side of the paralysis) cervicals, all toes, side of the neck, and reflexes to the affected areas.*

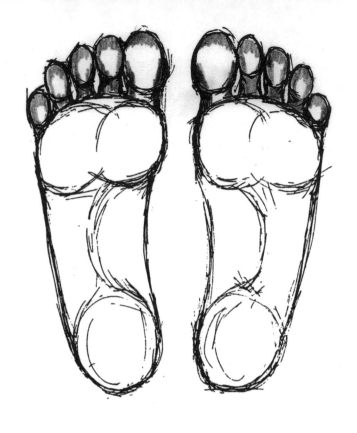

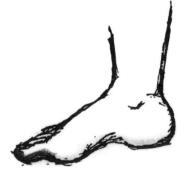 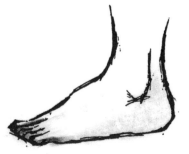

Page 6

## II. PARAPLEGIA

Definition: Paraplegia is defined as paralysis of the legs or lower part of the body.

Hank, the grandson of two of our regular clients, was visiting from another state. He was in his early twenties and was involved in an accident in his teens that left him paralyzed. He had been to several specialists, and was learning to live life as a paraplegic. Hank agreed to Reflexology therapy only to satisfy his grandmother. As his visit with them was for only ten days, we asked him to consent to Reflexology treatments daily. Before beginning the second treatment, I asked if he noticed anything different, he rolled his eyes as if to say, "Yeah, right!." He was a strong non-believer in Reflexology. After the third visit, again I asked if he noticed any changes or feeling in his body.

He said, "Not really."

"What do you mean not really?" I asked.

"Well", he said, "I always knew I had a sensation in my feet. I could never pin point exactly where it was. I now know that it's in my heel"

Hank may not have been excited, but I was ecstatic! The next day he felt tingles down the shin bone area of his legs. During the sixth treatment, he felt the tingles change into a fluttering-like feeling. At the seventh session, he said his feet were sweating profusely and that they hadn't sweated since his accident. After the eighth and final treatment, there was color change in the legs. He had noticed it while in the bath tub as he sponged his legs, as they

Page 7

changed from grayish to pinkish color. (You can tell that a woman is writing this by the colors described - pinkish, grayish, scarlet). I implored him to extend his visit, in order to receive more Reflexology treatments. His grandparents begged him also, but he left as planned. I did hear that his wife took a couple of Reflexology Seminars in order to try to help him. That was *frustration!*

When we practiced Reflexology on clients who were paraplegic, we found the following reflexes to be the most helpful: *whole spine, brain, leg/knee/hip reflex, sciatic reflex, and the outer fifth zone.*

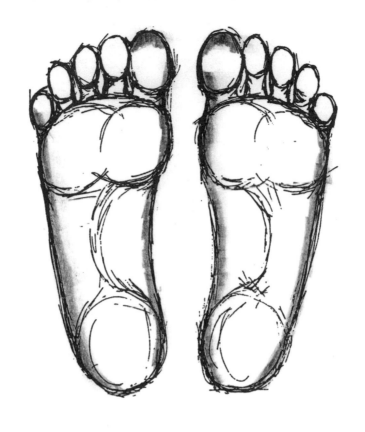

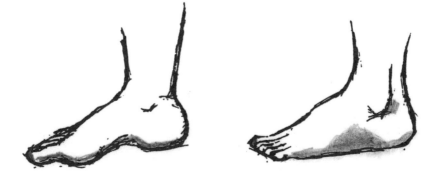

## III. LOU GEHRIG DISEASE, (AMYOTROPHIC LATERAL SCLEROSIS), A.L.S.

Definition: This is a progressive neuralgic disease, also called motor neuron disease. There is no known cause nor cure. Treatment is for providing relief, preventing complications, and maintaining optimal function as long as possible. The disease usually progresses rapidly, with death ensuing within an average of 2 to 5 years.

Many times our frustrations become success stories. We see results. Then something happens and the person doesn't continue with Reflexology and loses the progress that had been achieved. The following two stories are of success and frustration with A.L.S. (Amyotrophic Lateral Sclerosis).

(1) George. The first man, whom we will refer to as George, had been diagnosed four years earlier as having A.L.S. George had difficulty with his speech and one arm had become useless. He began receiving Reflexology therapy twice a week. Instantly, he had more energy and felt stronger. George had to travel fifty miles one way for his treatments. He had tried Reflexology before, and had found it to be relaxing, but not stimulating. Both Paul and I believe it is fine if there is slight discomfort during the therapy session. We enjoy saying, "No one sleeps in our chairs while we are in the room." However, we don't believe in brutality. There is a fine line between discomfort and pain. The level is different for each client. Initially, George received Reflexology treatments twice a week for three weeks. His progress was impressive. He no longer had difficulty speaking, and his arm didn't ache anymore. He was able to use his arm well enough to drive his car. He continued treatments once a week for three months. He felt

Reflexology gave him a new lease on life. As he was a Canadian and had to return home, we begged him to find a Reflexologist in Canada and to return to us for treatment as soon as possible. He found a Reflexologist who only relaxed him, and after a few treatments he stopped the visits. By the time he planned to return to Florida, he was too weak to drive. Also, his wife had become ill and unable to drive. George decided to remain in Canada, and within six months he died. *Frustration!*

(2) Bill. We watched the car pull into the office driveway. A women got out of the driver's side and went around the car to open the door for the passenger. The man was stooped over, nearly bent in half. He dragged his left leg as though he had suffered a stroke. Bill had been ill with A.L.S. for five years. His speech was so distorted that only his wife could understand him. They no longer socialized with others or went out for dinner. He could barely swallow and had trouble keeping food in his mouth. He didn't have control of his lips, drooling as he attempted a simple thing like trying to eat.

"Can we see him every day this week?" Paul asked. They agreed. After the first week, his wife was amazed at the improvement. Then she told us she was a nurse and had no idea what Reflexology could accomplish. His leg no longer dragged and his gait was almost normal. He was able to stand almost upright instead of being stooped and appearing to be bent in-half. Bill's energy level had increased greatly. This was after just one week of Reflexology therapy! He continued Reflexology treatments three times the second week. At the end of the second week, he was teary eyed when he told us that his daughter in Canada had telephoned them. She had cried with joy when Bill talked to her. It was the first time in more than a year that she could understand her father when he spoke. He continued regular treatments twice a week thereafter. His wife said they were now going out to dinner again. She had to cut his food into very small bites, but he was able to swallow and no longer did the food drip from his mouth. Bill had control. They were able to have marital relations again for the first time in two years. Everyone was happy! But it was time for him to go back home to Canada. He remained in fairly good health for four months. He passed away before he could return to Florida.

Reflexology did give him a better lifestyle for a short time. *Frustration!*

When we performed Reflexology treatments on clients with Lou Gehrig's disease, we found the following reflexes to be the most helpful: the *brain, whole spine, chest/lung, all glands, and the great toes.*

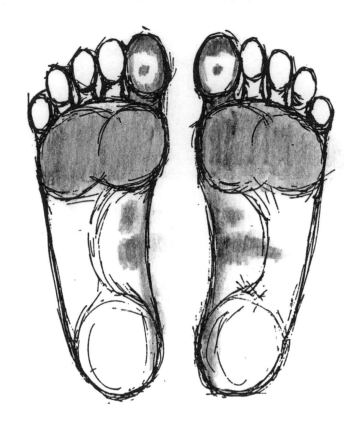

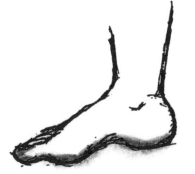 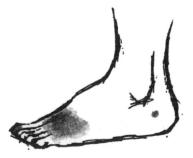

Page 14

# IV. CHRONIC FATIGUE IMMUNE DYSFUNCTION SYNDROME

Chronic means persisting for a long time. Fatigue is a state of increased discomfort and decreased efficiency and a general feeling of exhaustion.

(1) Becky. Becky was a beautiful woman in her early thirties, married, with three children, but she was dysfunctional with no energy. There were days she would accomplish absolutely nothing. Becky suffered from deep depression and had gained a great deal of weight in a very short time. We offered her our money-back guarantee. We asked for seven treatments close together. Becky agreed. Her pituitary reflex was not sensitive but the reflexes to all the other glands were very sensitive. Paul was able to achieve a response by working the pituitary reflex on her thumbs, but not the toes. After four treatments Becky suffered less depression and experienced an increased energy level. We felt we weren't reaching the pituitary reflex well enough. However, the fifth treatment was the real turning point. The pituitary reflex area was *very* sensitive in both great toes. Her progress was noticed by everyone around her. Becky continued Reflexology therapy twice a week for several weeks, and she was able to discontinue her antidepressants and other medications, (with her doctor's permission). She lost twenty pounds without dieting, because her glandular system was becoming balanced. Becky started her own floral and crafts business. After two months of Reflexology she was able to reduce the frequency of her treatments. She began coming for treatments once every other week for a month, then once every three weeks. Last year Becky and her family moved to another state and we were so afraid she would regress. She tried other Reflexologists (in her area) and was dissatisfied. Becky continues to work her own hands and the areas

*Page 15*

she can reach on her feet. She has remained healthy and no longer suffers from chronic fatigue syndrome. *Success!* Her plans are to take her first Reflexology Seminar this year. Becky feels she already knows more about Reflexology than the people claiming to be Reflexologists in her area. Her goal is to take the classes and prove that Reflexology works, as we proved it worked on her. We aren't saying that we are the only Reflexologists who get results. There are thousands of good qualified Reflexologists throughout the U.S. and all over the world. It's just a shame that there are unqualified people alluding to be Reflexologists that give the discipline a bad name.

(2) Emily. Emily was eighty years young. She still worked thirty hours a week as a hair stylist. One morning she awoke to find herself with absolutely no energy. She was unable to go to work. She became extremely depressed and went to her doctor that very same day. The doctor admitted her into the hospital for tests. Emily remained in the hospital for seven days with no definite diagnosis. The doctors finally agreed that Emily was suffering from Chronic Fatigue Immune Dysfunction Syndrome. Four months later she was still dysfunctional and on medication for her depression. When she came to our office for her first Reflexology therapy treatment she was in tears. She said, "I am eighty years old and feel it! I never thought this could happen to me. I have always been active physically and mentally. Something has to help me." Reflexology: the *Last Resort!* After her first three Reflexology treatments she began seeing some improved energy. It wasn't until the seventh treatment that her pituitary reflex was sensitive to pressure, and we began seeing great improvement. Emily's doctors lessened her depression medications, and believe it or not, within a month Emily was back to work. She was performing all activities she had been able to perform before she was diagnosed with

Chronic Fatigue Syndrome; and, furthermore, without any drugs or medication ! *Success!*


(3) Lee. Lee didn't know what was wrong with her. She would walk for several hours daily and attend many weekly Bible meetings. Suddenly she was homebound. Lee was willing to try Reflexology to see if she could regain her energy. Unlike the previous two cases of Chronic Fatigue Syndrome, Lee did not go through the tests to determine what was causing her sudden change in energy and the depression. After four Reflexology treatments, Lee began to notice a definite change in her depression level. All of her reflexes for the glandular system were sensitive; especially the pituitary reflex. It took only two weeks of Reflexology for her to gain enough energy to again attend all of her Bible classes. After a full month of Reflexology treatments, she had gained enough strength to be able to do her daily walking! *Success!*


(4) Sally. Not all cases produce quick results. Take Sally for instance; she had been under a doctor's care for twelve years. She was taking antidepressants and sleeping pills. She has two lovely children and a very loving husband. At the time of this writing, Sally has had twenty-five Reflexology Therapy treatments. She is sleeping without sleeping pills, and has asked her doctor to begin gradually reducing her antidepressants. Sally is improving at a slow but continual pace. Her thinking ability is much better and the pressure she was feeling in her head that made it hard for her to concentrate is gone. Her mood swings have lessened also.

Sally said, "I no longer have huge highs and lows, I only have light waves. I don't cry at the drop of a hat and I'm cooking meals once more. I didn't think there was hope for me until Reflexology."

Sally continues to receive two Reflexology Therapy treatments each week and is progressing nicely.

When we did Reflexololgy treatments on clients with Chronic Fatigue Immune Dysfunction we found the following reflexes to be the most helpful: *pituitary, pituitary, pituitary, adrenal, adrenal, adrenal, all glands, and the whole spine.*

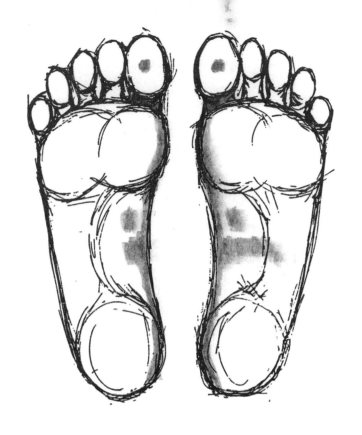

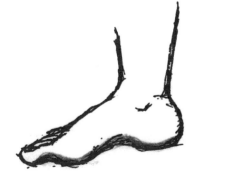 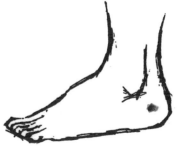

Page 19

# V. EMPHYSEMA

Definition:    This term is generally used to designate chronic pulmonary emphysema, a lung disorder in which the terminal bronchioles become plugged with mucus.

(1) Darrell.   We have two lovely sisters who come for regular Reflexology treatments twice a month. One has diabetes and the other one has circulation problems. Because Reflexology did help both of them, they encouraged their brother, Darrell, to try Reflexology for his problems with emphysema. He was leery at first, but he saw how much improved his sisters were since receiving regular Reflexology therapy, so he decided to try a few treatments. When he first came to our office his breathing was so labored that he was gasping for air, and he walked very slowly with great effort.   We asked for an initial three treatments close together, after which we would discuss whether or not he had experienced any improvement. Darrell had told us that his emphysema becomes chronic and that he is usually hospitalized two or three times a year with it. With each subsequent Reflexology treatment, he saw improvement. When the first three treatments were completed, Darrell  decided he wanted two treatments a week for a couple of weeks.   After the biweekly-weekly sessions,  he had improved enough to be able to receive treatments only  once a week. After one month of treatments, he was coming once every other week. How was Darrell  doing at this point?  He hung three ceiling fans in one day.  It had been years since he could hold his arms above his head.  He washed his car and mowed the lawn.  He was totally functional.  It has been three years since his last hospitalization for emphysema.  Darrell is on our video tape, because a local television station wanted to interview someone that had experienced good results with Reflexology. *Success?* Yes!

(2) Barbara. Barbara suffered from emphysema so drastically that she needed oxygen at all times. We found it necessary to make house calls twice a week for one month. She progressed to the point of being able to go off the oxygen for short periods of time. Once again, she was able to enjoy going out to restaurants. She would leave a portable oxygen tank in the car, in case she needed it. She continued her Reflexology treatments once a week for another month. We showed her husband how to perform the diaphragm relaxer technique. He also learned how to reduce the edema with Reflexology techniques on the chest/lung reflex area of her feet. This was the only method by which she could extend the treatments. That was four years ago. She is still doing fine.

(3) Lilly. Lilly has been receiving Reflexology treatments for more than ten years. She comes to our office once every three weeks. When Lilly first started with Reflexology, her emphysema had made it difficult for her to enjoy a meal in public. She would gasp for air and have severe coughing spells. Lilly felt improvement with each Reflexology treatment. She received six treatments in the first two weeks. Then she came for treatments once a week for an entire month. She was now able to go to the neighborhood doughnut shop for her daily cup of coffee and one doughnut. This was something she truly enjoyed doing each morning after she worked her crossword puzzle. She increases her treatments if the air is high with pollen; otherwise she maintains well with Reflexology every three weeks.

(4) Artie. Artie was a cigarette smoker for many years. Her emphysema was so advanced that she had been seeing her medical doctor every four to six weeks, for the past year. Artie received Reflexology treatments twice a week for three weeks. When she

went to her doctor he was so pleased with her improvement that her next appointment was made for three months later. The nurse could not believe it and even questioned the fact that Artie didn't need an appointment sooner. The doctor assured her that unless Artie had a problem, she did not need to come back for three months.

When we performed Reflexololgy on clients with Emphysema, we found the following reflexes to be the most helpful: *solar plexus, diaphragm, chest/lung, adrenals, lymphatic, and of course ileocecal.*

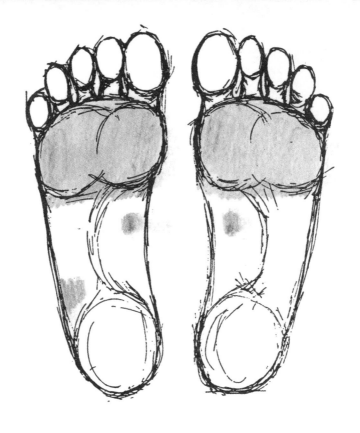

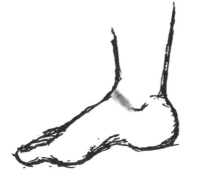

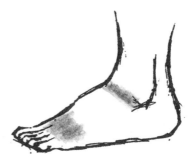

# VI. LEG PROBLEMS

Definition: This is a common complaint for a multitude of reasons. The clients may complain of: swelling, stiffness, aching, burning sensations, nervous twitching, numbness, lack of feeling, feeling like there is a tight band around the calf, etc.

(1) Thelma. Thelma was in her early seventies when she came to our office complaining of leg pains. Thelma's feet and legs were swollen and purple. The veins in her calves were raised and she had a lot of broken capillaries. She had been in this condition for fifteen years. Reflexology: her *Last Resort*. She could only wear a pair of specially made shoes with special supports. Even then, she could only walk a very short distance, such as from the car to the house. After her five initial treatments of Reflexology therapy she was able to walk without pain in her feet or legs. She received two treatments a week for two more weeks, and was able to wear some of her regular shoes. Thelma was so pleased with her success that she sent her husband, her son, her daughter, her son-in-law, and her grandson to our office to experience a Reflexology treatment! Referrals are your best form of advertisement! Achieve success as quickly as possible and you will see your clientele increase. *Success? Yes!*

(2) Ray. Ray came for his first Reflexology treatment at the age of ninety. The swelling in his legs and feet were balloon-like. He was unable to wear any shoes. His legs had several small sores which were extremely discolored. Reflexology may well have been Ray's *Last Resort*. His legs and feet felt like solid wood. It was very difficult to give him a Reflexology treatment, because we had to work almost the entire session just to reduce some of the

extreme edema. He received Reflexology twice a week for three weeks before the swelling remained lessened until the next treatment. Progress was slow, but progressive. Within two months, Ray's legs were half the size they had been before his Reflexology therapy. He continued treatments twice a month. He was able to wear shoes and walk two blocks to the neighborhood diner for dinner, without discomfort. Ray is now ninety two and doing well. *Success!*

(3) Earle. Earle was eighty years old when he first came to our office. His legs were the color of deep purple and there were ulcers on the right calf. He was the poorest looking excuse for a man you could imagine. He was not clean! In order to work him, I had to apply corn starch to his feet so the caked-on muck didn't get under my nails and his odor almost made me sick. It was nearly impossible to give him a good Reflexology treatment. When Earle left the office, I never expected to see him again. Was I ever wrong! A few weeks after his first Reflexology treatment, he called for another appointment. I sprayed my room so that I wouldn't smell his body odor. Again, I dusted his feet heavily with corn starch. Why didn't I wash his feet? I'm not a pedicurist, a podiatrist, nor a nurse. I'm not qualified according to the health department to bathe someone, not even their feet. It's not a part of Reflexology! After the second treatment, he wanted to schedule a series of treatments. I tried to be tactful and suggested that he help me get faster results.

"How?" he asked.

"By soaking your feet in *hot* water the night before your appointment," I replied. (Attempting to be tactful.)

"What can I soak them in?" he asked.

I looked at the dirty, crusted legs and replied, "The bath tub?

His reply shocked me! " Oh, I can't use the bath tub," he said, "that's where I store my newspapers."

I thought to myself, "When was the last time you bathed? " From that time on, I handed him  baby wipes to use on his feet and lower legs before the treatments. After a few times, his feet weren't too bad to work. Earle received Reflexology treatments three times a week for two weeks. His ulcers had healed and he insisted he now only needed Reflexology twice a month.   In our conversations, I was shocked to find that he had donated  $10,000 to our local hospital, and $5,000 to an Indian reservation! He was generous to others, but he would not spend the money on himself.   Earle needed weekly if not twice weekly Reflexology treatments   to improve his blood supply in the lower limbs.  He would only make Reflexology appointments for every other week.  When he passed away,  the  cause  of  death  was  *poor  circulation.*   ***Imagine!*** ***Frustration!***


(4) Tess.  Tess came to our office walking with a cane.  When she sat down in the chair, I proceeded to remove her right shoe and knee-high nylon.  I placed my left hand on her left leg and was ready to remove her left shoe, when I felt the lack of circulation beneath my hand on her leg.  I thought, "My goodness this lady needs circulation; I have never felt such a dead feeling leg." The expression on my face must have changed, because she asked me if I was all right.   After smiling at her and assuring her that I was fine, she asked me to please leave her left shoe on, because it was attached to her prosthesis.   No wonder it didn't feel normal. Foolish me! Tess was able to improve her blood and nerve supply with Reflexology therapy treatments.

(5) Stan. Stan was a carpenter by trade. There was nothing he couldn't build. Stan's problem was that his legs didn't want to support him. Stan complained that his calves felt hard and solid, yet they didn't feel strong enough to support his body weight. He could no longer climb a ladder without his legs giving way. He had to quit work at the early age of sixty. He was devastated and bored to tears. His son suggested that he try Reflexology. With each Reflexology treatment, Stan felt his legs improve. He was working again in just two weeks. We met a friend of Stan's at the city licensing department. When the gentleman discovered that we were Reflexologists, he commented, "My friend tried Reflexology and I know how much it helped him. Why, he is even back to full time work. I have told a lot of people with leg problems to try Reflexology." *Success!*

When we did Reflexology on clients with leg complaints, the following reflexes were found to be the most helpful: *hip/knee/leg, lumbar/sacral, groin, hip/sciatic, pelvic, lymphatic and the entire fifth zone on the plantar of the foot.*

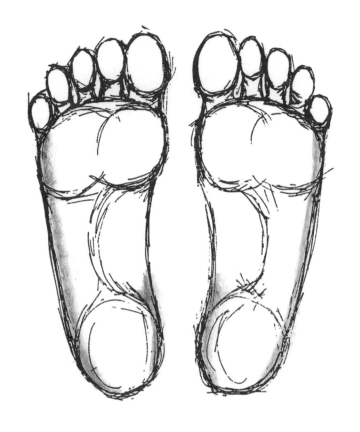

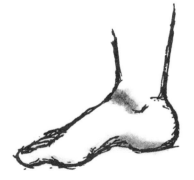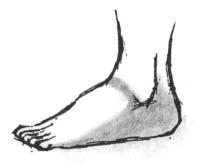

Page 28

# VII. RESTLESS LEG SYNDROME

Definition: Unpleasant deep discomfort inside the calves when sitting or lying down, especially before sleep, causing an irresistible urge to move the legs.

Paul and I have clients coming to us with varied complaints that are not directly related to back pain. Yet, when working the feet the most sensitive areas are the hip, sciatic or low back reflexes.

(1) Frank. This was true with Frank. He suffered from restless leg syndrome. The following are his words written in 1990: " I am a 72 year old male and have had this problem for over 40 years. I have been to 55 medical doctors and the best hospitals in Philadelphia, Pa., and have had all types of tests, scans, etc., but no one could help me."

He goes on to describe his condition. "I would get up three or four times every single night, walk the floor and rub my legs. There was no peace, even relaxing in a chair would bring on the condition. I tried all types of doctor's prescribed medications, sedatives and vitamins, but to no avail."

Frank decided to try Reflexology as his *Last Resort.* His letter goes on to explain what Reflexology treatments did for him. "This method helps relax tension, improves blood and nerve supply, also helps nature to normalize. The fifth treatment showed I was getting results."

After each treatment he saw further progress. He has been a regular client since 1990. He and his wife have depended on Reflexology for many problems through the years, but no longer for restless leg syndrome. *Success!*

(2) Chad.   Chad's wife learned about Reflexology from a co-worker.  She had told her co-worker how concerned she was about Chad's restless legs.  Chad would keep her up much of the night with his constant thrashing or shaking of his legs, and getting up to walk.   Chad came to our office and received five consecutive Reflexology treatments.  He and his wife could not believe the difference in his restless legs.  He was able to sleep through the night and had only slight discomfort.   Chad continued with Reflexology Therapy once a week for the remainder of the month. Chad is a regular once a month maintenance client, who no longer has any signs of restless legs. *Success!*


(3) Keith.  Keith was visiting from Ontario, Canada.  His neighbor at the mobile park where he was staying was very concerned about Keith's sleepless nights due to his restless legs.  The neighbor recommended Reflexology Therapy.  Also, Keith was  a diabetic and the circulation in his legs and feet were extremely poor.  The neighbor finally talked Keith into coming to the office and told him of our money-back guarantee.   After Keith received five Reflexology treatments every other day, he was a firm believer in Reflexology.  He was only in Florida for one month.  After his initial five treatments, he received Reflexology twice a week the next week, then once a week until he returned to Canada.  His restless legs never bothered him again after the seventh Reflexology treatment. *Success!*

When we performed Reflexology on a client with restless leg syndrome we found the following reflexes to be the most helpful: *hip/knee/leg, lumbar, hip/sciatic, pelvic area, groin and the entire outer fifth zone on the plantar.*

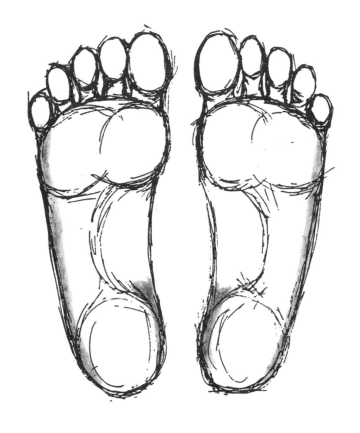

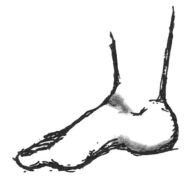 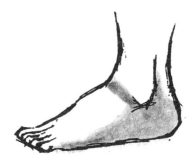

Gage 31

# VIII.  SCIATIC AND LOW BACK PAIN

Definition:   The sciatic is a nerve extending from the base of the spine down the thigh, with branches throughout the lower leg and foot.   Inflammation of the sciatic nerve causes pain along its course.

Almost everyone at sometime has complained about low back pain or sciatic discomfort.   Results are usually rapid with Reflexology treatments.   In most of the usual cases the client feels some improvement after the first treatment.   We also like to show them which reflexes they can work on their hands to help achieve faster results.

There are times when people come to us complaining of foot pain. Either the foot is burning or the side of the foot aches severely. When working the reflexes on the feet, many times it is still the hip, sciatic, or low lumbar reflexes that show the most sensitivity. After working the sensitivity out, the original complaint no longer exists.

(1) Jay.   Paul and I had worked all week in our offices, and on Friday we traveled from St. Petersburg to Ft. Lauderdale, assisting in teaching an Original Ingham Method of Reflexology Seminar. We traveled back home late Sunday evening, totally exhausted. After unpacking the car we retrieved our phone messages.   One was a frantic message for help.   The women said her husband was suffering with back spasms.   He had fallen off a ladder early Saturday morning. We returned her call, to see if it was still necessary for us to see her husband. We could hear his screams over the phone.   We went over to his home immediately.   Paul worked on the man's feet for one-half hour, then I worked his feet for one half hour.   We continued to alternate like this until after midnight.   Jay had even placed a cloth in his mouth to stifle the

screams when the spasms recurred. The spasms were often, about every four minutes. Jay had been in this condition since the fall on Saturday morning. Neither Paul nor I had experienced "working" someone in such pain. By midnight the spasms had lessened and he was able to sleep. I can't explain how exhausted and drained we were. Jay was not an easy client to work. He had what Reflexologists might call tough feet to work. It took as much pressure as we could give to achieve any lasting results. We have never performed Reflexology on anyone as diligently or for such an extended period of time as we did Jay due to the toughness of his feet. In the morning he was able to walk and use the restroom for the first time during the entire weekend. His doctors advised him to have back surgery, but Jay is postponing surgery and using alternative methods. He has been able to do this for more than five years, as of this writing.


(2) Jack. The most unusual sciatica case we have had was a young man, who called our office and said he had been on the living-room floor, flat on his back for the entire weekend. His mother-in-law insisted that he get help. He wanted to know if I only worked one leg, could he get half price. "What? Of course not! I tried to explain that it is not possible to work only one foot and get the needed results. I said, "I can't work only one foot and get the results you need." He then explained that he had only one foot. I said, I would work his hands and one foot, and if he would allow me, I would work the stump of the other leg as well. During the session, Jack explained how he had lost his leg, his job, and his wife in less than three months. All of that had happened just two years ago. We started the treatment on his hands and then his right foot. His stump was very close to the groin, so I left the pant leg tucked and worked over the material and not directly on the skin. When "working" on the stump, it would jump straight up, and I would have to hang on. Jack had no control over it; the stump was

spastic. After working Reflexology on the stump for five or six minutes, the stump calmed and Jack had a feeling of warmth in it. He said that he could feel both the circulation improve and the energy in the stump. After just one Reflexology treatment, Jack had no more pain in his back. Jack continues to receive Reflexology for his circulation and muscle tonement to the stump.

(3) Don.   Don was homebound for two weeks before calling our office. He had seen several medical practitioners and was told his pain was coming from his hip. His neighbor pleaded with him to try Reflexology treatment before considering surgery. When Don arrived at our office, he was very bent over and walking with two canes. He could not straighten up and he said he was in constant pain. After his first treatment Paul felt Reflexololgy should ease his pain. We weren't sure as to what level, or if treatments would help the hip condition.   Paul offered Don our money-back guarantee, if he would receive Reflexology treatments every day for five days. Don was a non-believer in Reflexology. "How could anyone touch my feet and help my back or hip?" he asked. "Money back? I have nothing to lose and everything to gain. Do what you have to do," he said.

The pain in the reflex areas to the chronic sciatic nerve, hip, leg and knee were more painful than the condition with which he was suffering. Not until the fourth treatment did he feel less discomfort in the reflex areas. After one week, Don was able to fly to Las Vegas and walk anywhere he wished without pain. That was five months ago.   He receives Reflexology every few weeks as maintenance. *Success!*

(4) Paul. My husband is a classic example of back pain. When remodeling our house, he attempted to move an upper wall cabinet

unit, and the entire unit fell from the wall onto his shoulders. He felt as if his spine had compressed and he experienced instant pain. There was no one at home at the time to help him. Paul was forced to continue to hold the entire eight foot upper wall cabinet unit on his shoulders until he could get it outside. There was no room for him to maneuver it in the kitchen. He struggled for what seemed like an eternity before he somehow managed to get the unit out of the house. When I arrived home later that evening, Paul was unable to move as the pain was unbearable. I gave him Reflexology Therapy immediately and then continued to work his feet for one half-hour every hour for several hours. Paul slept through the night. The next day he was able to walk, but there were times when the muscles would spasm causing great pain. Sometimes the pain would stop him in his steps. With each Reflexology treatment he received immediate relief, but the relief wasn't lasting. Paul received several treatments daily for a full week before relief was continual. It took several weeks before he was back to normal. If we had not been true believers in Reflexology we would have racked up some serious medical bills, as Paul had seriously injured himself.

(5) Diane. I, too, have had to rely on Reflexology to ease back pain. I was visiting my sister in up-state New York. We had all been enjoying her hot tub. Our hot tub at home has a raised decking around it, but my sister's tub sits on a low deck. Like most people, I am a creature of habit. While I was talking with my sister, who was standing on the raised deck near the hot tub area, I lifted my leg to step out of the tub. The next thing I knew; I was on my back wedged between the lower and upper decks. I screamed for them not to touch me. I thought I had broken my back or my ribs. I finally got my breath and felt that I was to the point where I could be moved. Paul helped me into the house. It was wonderful that Paul knew Reflexology, because he worked my feet until I fell asleep. I' m not sure how long it took, but it must have been several

hours. I slept flat on my back. When I awoke the pain was excruciating; it wouldn't allow me to roll over or move. Paul got out of bed and immediately began to work on my feet. After a fifteen minute Reflexology treatment I was able to get out of bed. Paul had to dress me, because I didn't have any flexibility in my back. My family wanted me to go to the hospital. I reasoned that if my ribs were cracked they don't really do anything except give you pain pills. I had taken a laxative the night before to insure I would know if there was any internal bleeding. Everything seemed fine. My ribs hurt, breathing was difficult, and I was badly bruised. As Reflexologists, we know what results are possible. Each treatment temporarily eased the pain. It took daily treatments for a week in order to achieve a degree of comfort. As I look back, I probably did bruise my ribs, because the discomfort when laughing or sneezing lasted for a few months. Today I am fine.


(6) Tom. Tom had back surgery three years prior to his Reflexology therapy treatment. The surgery left him with a noticeable limp. He could not stand up straight. The doctors told him that this was as good as he was ever going to be. After three Reflexology treatments, he was able to stand up straight and had only a slight limp. Tom received another two treatments before seeing the full results of no limping and straight posture.

(7) Tandy. Recovering alcoholics have a very difficult time if they are in pain. Tandy was a young lady attending AA meetings and doing very well. She had been a drug user and an alcoholic. This meant that she could not afford to take any pain pills to ease her back pain. Tandy had a chronic back disorder that could put her flat on her back without warning. Instead of medication she received Reflexology to ease her pain when her back would flare up. She once stated, "I don't know what I would do or how I could

live without Reflexology to eliminate my back pain." Reflexology was and will continue to be her *Last Resort.*

When we did Reflexology therapy on clients complaining of low back or sciatic pain, we found the following reflexes to be the most helpful: *hip/sciatic, hip/leg/knee, pelvic area, chronic sciatic, lumbar, fifth zone of the plantar, shoulder, and cervicals.*

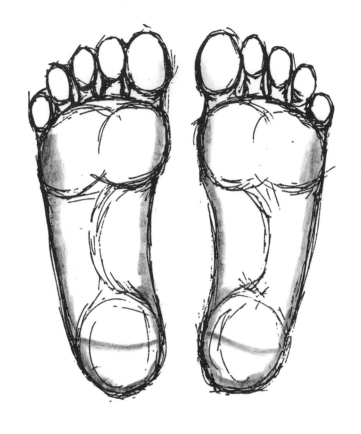

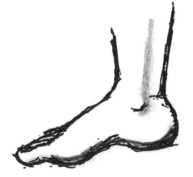

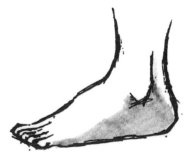

# IX. DIABETES

Definition: Diabetes is a general term referring to a variety of disorders characterized by excessive urination, hyperglycemia and glycosuria. It is the result of inadequate production or utilization of insulin.

We have practiced Reflexology therapy on many diabetics. One man no longer needs injections and his doctor prescribes only a small amount of medication for his maintenance. Many diabetics have poor circulation, especially in the lower extremities. With Reflexology, we see great improvement in their feet and legs where there once had been poor circulation.

(1) Dolly. Dolly was an eighty-old diabetic, who smoked heavily. Her great toes were black and all of her small toes were gray. There was seepage coming from her right great toe because of an open sore at the tip of the toe. She had already seen a surgeon and he scheduled vascular surgery in two weeks. Before we started her Reflexology therapy treatment, we gave Dolly a bandage to put on the sore. We were extremely careful to stay away from the injured area. We concentrated on the base of the great toe and worked all of her little toes. The second Reflexology treatment showed that her sore had formed a large, thick scab. The doctor had given her ointment, so we had her to put the ointment on a bandage and again cover the sore. The gray color of her small toes had already changed to a lighter shade of gray. We suggested that Dolly come to the office every other day. By the third treatment, the sore on her great toe seemed almost healed. While working her little toes during the third treatment, there was a sudden release of poison like green liquid from under one of her small toe nails that propelled across the room. The following treatment showed her small toes to look pink and healthy, rather than the original gray.

The great toes were no longer black and the sore on the great toe had completely healed. After her fifth treatment, Dolly went back to the surgeon for her scheduled appointment. He looked at her feet and asked, "What did you do? Stop smoking?" She told him she had received Reflexology treatments. He just shook his head and told her, "You don't need me anymore. You can go back to your regular physician." No surgery was needed. *Success!*

(2) Paula.    Another diabetic client who had surgery for a hip replacement and complained of poor circulation. Paula was eighty-two years old when she received her first Reflexology treatment. We gave her treatments twice a week for two weeks. There was great improvement in the color and circulation of her legs; furthermore, she had no more discomfort from her hip and knee. About one month after her first Reflexology treatment, her doctor allowed her to reduce her medication for diabetes. Finally, she didn't need any medication. Her blood tests now indicate that she's in excellent physical condition. She decided to continue with the Reflexology treatments for overall good health twice a month. She still takes no medication and is in good health at the age of eighty-nine years young.

(3) Henry. Henry had been diagnosed with diabetes. He was complaining that feelings in his feet were nearly gone and the circulation in his legs was very poor. When Henry first came to our office for Reflexology, he only knew Reflexology might help him regain some feeling in his feet. He told us, "Yesterday, I dressed and put my shoes on to go to the bank. I began searching the house for the car keys. I searched everywhere imaginable, but I could not find them. A few hours later my wife came home and she began searching for the keys. No keys were found. I decided to take a rest or a short nap, so I removed my shoes to lie down. I couldn't believe it!   Both my house and car keys were in my shoe!   I was

walking on them and couldn't even feel them. It could have been something sharp, I would have bled and would never have felt it. I'm here for help." Reflexology - the *Last Resort!* His first three Reflexology treatments were easy. We worked his feet with great pressure since he couldn't feel the pressure nor the reflexes in the feet. By the fourth session, he experienced great discomfort during his treatment, even with our applying light pressure to his feet. He said, "I'll never again say I can't feel it when you work my reflexes. I can feel everything you are doing." After six Reflexology therapy treatments, Henry had excellent feeling return to his feet. Also, the redness that had been present on his feet had disappeared. His legs felt better, but he still needed more treatments for the necessary results. Henry went back to Ontario, Canada and continued his Reflexology treatments there. *Success!*


(4) Tom. Tom was a diabetic with poor circulation. I remember the first time he came to the office. Someone in the office asked us if he was terminal. His coloring was gray and he looked like the walking dead. His legs were black in some areas and there were little thin skinned bubbles along the veins. Tom received Reflexology treatments three times a week two weeks before we saw much improvement. His coloring had improved, his legs were getting better texture and he felt stronger than he had in over a year. He continued the treatments twice a week for a month. His entire family received at least one Reflexology treatment after seeing Tom was so much better. His legs were now a light brown and most of the bubbles had disappeared. He was able to return to work after three weeks of Reflexology treatments. Tom would be the first to tell you that Reflexology was *his Last Resort* and that it works!

(5) Carol. Carol is a very sweet older lady who came to our office with swollen, purple legs. She would become dizzy when

standing, and couldn't walk for any length of time. She was seventy-seven years old when she began Reflexology. Today she is eighty years young and continues to receive Reflexology therapy once a week. Getting rid of the swelling was easier than effecting color change in the calves. After just three treatments, she was no longer dizzy when standing, and didn't bump into walls when walking down a hallway. *Success!* I recall one visit when Carol came for her usual Reflexology treatment and complained about loss of appetite. She was usually weak, because she couldn't force herself to eat. We asked if her doctor had changed any of her medications. She replied that he had changed her thyroid medication. We suggested she call her doctor and tell him how she felt and ask if the change in medication could be causing the new problem. Carol, like so many others, didn't want to call him or bother him. Because she already had an appointment set up in two weeks. Carol decided to wait until the appointment. The following week when she came in for her regular Reflexology treatment she was in such a weakened state that she was unable to drive. She had to have a friend bring her to our office and even help her walk. We begged her not to wait another week until her next scheduled doctor appointment. Finally, she agreed to call her doctor that very day. Her medication was changed and so was she. Now, she is active with friends, shopping, dining, and giving dinner parties! She walks for one hour three or four times a week and receives Reflexology therapy one hour every week.


(6) Hans. A local medical doctor asked us to visit a man who had an ulcerated wound on his calf due to diabetes and poor circulation. The doctor was administering chelation therapy and felt Reflexology would also be a complementary therapy. The wound was six inches long and two and a half inches wide. Neither Paul nor I had ever seen a more seriously ulcerated sore. Staying away from the open area of the wound, I began doing

Reflexology on the feet, slightly above the ankle. I worked to soften the tight tissue surrounding the wound in hopes of improving the circulation to the total area. Three house calls a week for two weeks were made. The healing was progressing and it appeared Hans would not need an amputation. As his circulation began to improve the level of discomfort during his Reflexology treatments increased. We understand that when circulation improves it is not always comfortable for the client. Think of a leg that goes to sleep and when it awakens it is not very pleasant. Hans continued to complain about the discomfort no matter how gentle the treatment. I began to think, "Maybe it's because it's a woman who is causing him discomfort and that it bothers him." I suggested Paul "work" on him the next time and he agreed. Paul was super gentle but the man refused to put up with *any* discomfort. Hans decided to stop his Reflexology treatments. We heard three months later his leg was amputated. (Sounds like discomfort to me.) Hans suffered a stroke after leg surgery and is in a nursing home, as of this writing. Reflexology was helping him, it might have saved his leg if he had been more patient. *Frustration!*

(7) Ron. We were asked by a client to make a house call to see a man who had been a diabetic for many years. Ron's circulation had become so poor that amputation of the foot was necessary. We gave him three Reflexology treatments the first week and he saw some improvement. There was feeling in his ankle and some feeling in the feet. Reflexology was *his Last Resort.* When feeling began to return there was discomfort. He needed Reflexology, but he refused. We stopped to see him a week later and could not believe what we saw. He was sitting at the kitchen table and under his one foot there was a puddle of water. The fluid was coming from his foot. That very week his foot was amputated. Two weeks later the leg was removed from the knee down. Shortly after that, they removed the leg to the upper thigh. Too many

surgeries too close together and his heart couldn't take it. He suffered a severe heart attack and subsequently died. *Frustration!*


(8) Rob. Rob came for his first Reflexology treatment at the age of ninety. He could not find any shoes to fit him; due to the swelling in his legs and feet. On his legs were several small sores which were extremely discolored. He received Reflexology twice a week for three weeks. The results were that the swelling in his legs and feet became half the size they had been before Reflexology therapy. He continued with Reflexology treatments once a week for another month and was able to wear shoes and walk two blocks without discomfort. The reason we know that he was able to walk two blocks is because Rob hates to cook and there is a neighborhood diner two blocks away from his home. Rob is thankful that he is able to walk again. It had been his practice to walk to the diner nightly. *Success!*

(9) Martin. I watched as a new client got out of his car and walked toward the office door. He shuffled his feet like Tim Conway does when he impersonates an old man. Martin said that his legs felt like two-by-fours, solid and hard. He had been a special helper for elementary school children with math problems. Martin was devastated when he had to stop, because he could not walk from his handicapped parking area to his room at the school. Martin was seventy-six years old when he received his first Reflexology treatment. After three Reflexology treatments, Martin was able to lift his feet when he walked, and his knees were once again bending. When it came time for the new school year to begin, Martin was there in fine spirits, walking with no difficulty at all. He worked at school until he was eighty-four years old. Reflexololgy was his *Last Resort.*

(10) Doc. Doc is a local Dentist that suffers from diabetes. When Doc first came to our office he had a cast on his right lower leg and foot. He had had some corrective surgery to his right foot. His left leg was very swollen and contained a great deal of fluid. He had previously had several toes removed on both feet. His main complaint now was the ulcerated wounds on the plantar of both feet. Doc came for Reflexology treatments three times  the first week. His left leg became a normal size and the edema was no longer a problem. His ulcers were  healing nicely and it was time for his cast to be removed. After the cast was removed the task of getting the swelling  down in his right leg was not an easy one. Paul had to use a great deal of pressure to achieve the desired results.  Doc is now wearing  regular shoes for the first time in several months.  He continues with his Reflexology treatments twice a week to continue to improve his blood supply.


When we did Reflexology to clients that were diabetics, we found the following reflexes to be the most helpful:  *pancreas, liver, adrenals, pituitary and all glands.  If there is edema add lymph/groin.*

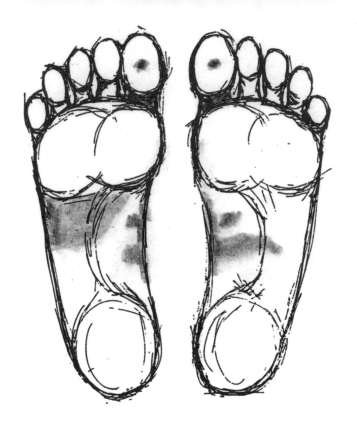

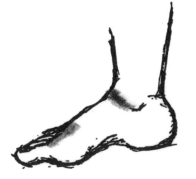 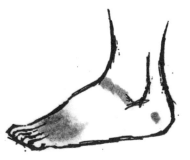

Page 46

# X. CARPAL TUNNEL SYNDROME

Definition: This is a symptom resulting from the compression of the median nerve in the carpal tunnel of the wrist. This can cause pain and burning or sometimes tingling in the fingers and hand, even extending to the elbows.

(1) Debra. Debra is an international concert pianist. She was diagnosed as having carpal tunnel syndrome in her right wrist. She was suffering so much that she canceled her upcoming tour. The thought of surgery frightened her; especially, since there were no guarantees of success. The long recovery time would mean even more cancellations. When Debra wasn't on tour, she taught piano to many students at both the local college and her home. She could not give up her entire livelihood. Reflexology was *her Last Resort*. Debra came to the office and received five consecutive Reflexology treatments. We worked the wrists, the ankles, the hands and feet. The results were rapid. She has never canceled another concert because of carpal tunnel pain. Debra receives Reflexology therapy once a month. If she has any aches in her wrist, or is preparing for an upcoming concert, she immediately adds an extra Reflexology session. *Success!*

(2) Martha. Martha is a writer and a school teacher. She was diagnosed as having carpal tunnel syndrome in both wrists. She tried medication, injections and physical therapy. Surgery was prescribed. She didn't want to undergo surgery. She had one more year before retirement and she could not afford the time off from work that the surgery would require. Reflexology was *her Last Resort.* That was eight years ago. The first few Reflexology treatments showed her reflexes to the neck and cervical reflexes to be extremely sensitive. After three treatments the first week, Martha's pain was gone! Most clients return for Reflexology treatments for overall good health after seeing beneficial results. We still see this lady every few weeks.

(3) Don. Don, an executive with a large corporation, had pain when moving his right middle and ring fingers. He had already undergone surgery on his left hand and wrist. He wasn't willing to go through another surgery. When his Reflexology treatments began, he could not make a fist with either hand. After receiving treatments three times a week for two weeks Don could make a fist with both hands and there was no more pain in either his hands or wrists. He receives Reflexology therapy every other month. We let our clients decide when to come back for treatments. Personally, we can't imagine going more than two weeks without Reflexology. However, we must remember we don't have to pay for it either. Paul and I just "work" on each other!

When we did Reflexology to clients with Carpal Tunnel Syndrome, we found the following reflexes to be the most helpful: *cervicals, thoracic, and the neck/shoulder. (also the wrist and ankle)*

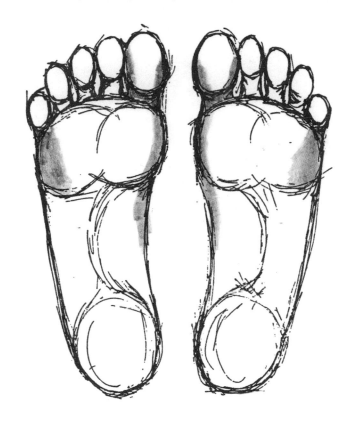

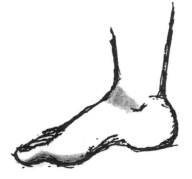

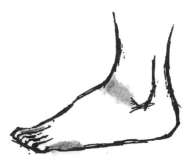

Page 49

# XI. TIC DOULOUREUX

Definition: This is a painful disorder involving the fifth cranial nerve. It is characterized by severe pain in the face and forehead on the affected side. The pain can be triggered by cold drafts, chewing, drinking cold liquids, brushing one's hair or teeth, or even washing the face. The following are three case studies of clients who had been diagnosed as having Tic Douloureux.

(1) Denise. These are Denise's own words taken from a letter she wrote to us in 1987. "I have had Tic Douloureux since 1969. I have tried everything. First, I was administered alcohol shots for three to four months. I tried acupuncture at the cost of $3000. It didn't help either." After that she had three radio frequency laser procedures. The letter continues, "I have had two surgical procedures, one for each side of my face. Four or five months following the last surgical procedure, the severe pains started again on my left side. My doctor said there was nothing more he could do but that I should keep taking the Dilantin medication. A few months ago, a friend told me about Reflexology. By that time, I could not talk or chew food or smile without getting extreme pain. I had nothing to lose and everything to gain, so I decided to try Reflexology." *Her Last Resort!* "The first week I had three treatments. The second week I had two treatments. The sharp pains ceased after the second week of Reflexology treatments. I haven't had any "stings" for over three weeks now, and I haven't taken any dilantin during those three weeks. " She has continued to receive Reflexology therapy every other week, and has remained pain free from Tic Douloureux.

(2) Fran.  The second client with Tic Douloureux would cover her entire face if there was any cold air or draft present.  She carried a wool scarf with her, even in Florida, since even in Florida in winter we sometimes experience  cold drafts.  She, too, experienced pain when brushing her hair, chewing, or washing her face.  Fran came to our office complaining of  knee problems and on her questionnaire she listed Tic Douloureux as a present ailment.  She was not on the same medications, or in constant pain, as our previous client, Denise.  We were able to maintain lack of pain more easily.  After administering Reflexology treatments to her twice a week for two weeks nothing brought the pain on except the cold drafts.  She could brush her hair, chew and wash her face without any discomfort.  Reflexology works. *Success!*

(3) Kathy.  Kathy was  not as advanced in the disease as the previously mentioned two clients.  She only suffered if she got in a cold draft, but had no problems when chewing, smiling or brushing her hair.  When she did have pain, the pain would last for at least the remainder of that day and sometimes for a few days more.  After five Reflexology sessions, she rarely had any flair ups, and when she did, it wasn't severe pain but only discomfort.  She continued Reflexology once a month for the remainder of her life-- some 10 years.

When we did Reflexology on clients suffering from Tic douloureux, we found the following reflexes to be the most helpful: *cervicals, great toe, neck, diaphragm, and  all toes*.

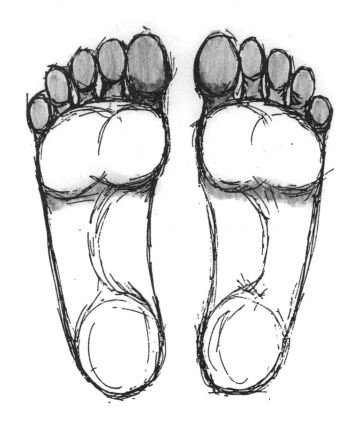

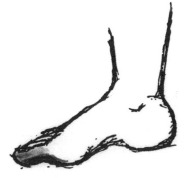
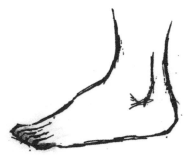

Page 52

# XII. HEEL SPURS

Definition: Spurs are formed by a mineral buildup on the calcaneus bone in the heel of the foot.

(1) June. Most Reflexologists can give examples of eliminating a heel spur with Reflexology treatments. June came to our office on two crutches. She couldn't wear shoes. She had a heel spur on both her feet. June had read an article in a magazine listing different alternative methods. Even though she was not familiar with Reflexology she was willing to try anything. The doctor had given her two injections of cortisone, resulting in little help. Her choices were Reflexology or surgery. Those choices made Reflexology her *Last Resort*. Her first Reflexology treatment was for one full hour, working both feet completely. When she stood up to go she did not need the crutches. She had fifteen minute Reflexology treatments daily on each heel for seven days. At the end of one week she was shopping at the flea market with no discomfort! That was nine years ago and the spurs have never given her anymore trouble.

(2) Fred. Fred was an active man in his early sixties. He was playing tennis four times a week, when he suddenly felt the pain of a heel spur. One of Fred's tennis buddies had had success with a heel spur from Reflexology therapy, so Fred came to our office. He wasn't very happy with the discomfort he felt when I worked the heel area and the spur. When he returned for the second treatment, he handed me a page which was ripped from a pornography magazine. I was shocked! He had seemed so nice. I thought, "Why would he hand me this filth?" My face must have been red because Fred laughed at my expression.

He said, "I thought you might want to redecorate your room with whips and chains." He considered my room to be a torture chamber. Working on spurs is <u>not pleasant.</u> Fred only needed three Reflexology sessions to eliminate all discomfort from his heel spur. *(P.S. He was a very nice man with a great sense of humor.)*


(3) Amber. I had just had my hair styled at the Gallerie of Hair Design when Mary, the owner of the salon, asked me to wait. Mary is a client of ours and knew Reflexology could help one of her other customers, so she wanted to introduce us. Mary explained that Amber had been suffering from heel spurs for five months. Amber already had had two injections of cortisone in both heels, resulting in little relief. Her first Reflexology treatment was a complete one hour session. Her left heel felt much better after the first treatment. She returned every day for four days to receive a fifteen minute Reflexology treatment on just her right heel. She had absolutely no more discomfort from spurs. Here is proof, again, that word of mouth is your best advertisement.

When we did Reflexology on clients with spurs, we found the following reflexes to be the most helpful: *heel, parathyroid, and all glands*.

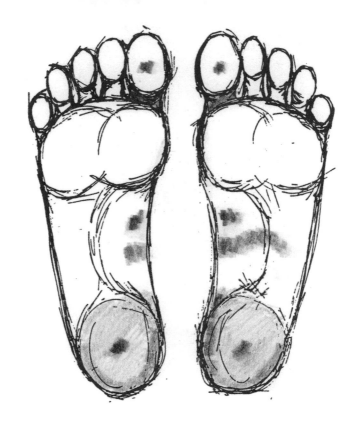

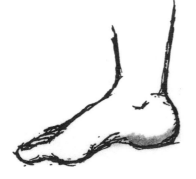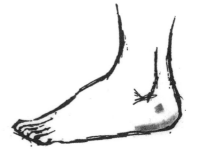

Page 65

# XIII. CHILDREN

I love little feet. Mothers have always loved their children's feet. One of the first things that some mothers do when returning home with her little ones is take off their shoes and socks and play with their tiny feet as well as clapping them together or playing stretch the leg to their nose "Phew! Stinky feet." How about playing "this little piggy?" Perhaps playing with their tiny toes helps their sinus reflexes. Most moms have kissed their children's feet and even held them to their cheeks. Yes, I love children's little feet!

As I was working my grandson, Jared's feet, he complained that I was hurting him. The reflex areas to the low lumbar and pelvic region were swollen. I used less pressure but continued his treatment. I explained that I had to work the soreness out. He trusted me. This is the grandchild that may very well become a good Reflexologist in the future. He loves Reflexology and believes in it. I asked him if he had "wiped-out" on his bike. "No," he answered.

I asked if he had fallen. "No." he said.

By the time I had worked out the tenderness on one foot and was going to the other foot he exclaimed, "I remember! I fell off the top of the slide."

I often wonder what children do during the day that might make them miserable at bed-time. Falling from the top of a slide might hurt a child but he or she might not remember the incident. Wouldn't it be ideal if every child received a brief foot Reflexology session when being tucked-in at night? Maybe that would eliminate some of the spankings that occur before bedtime.

A mother brought her two-month-old child into the office to see if Reflexology could help unplug the baby's tear duct, which had been plugged since birth. There was no way we could charge for a one hour treatment on feet so small. The first treatment was for about fifteen minutes. We instructed the mother how to "work" the necessary reflexes for best results. Between the mother working the baby often, and our doing Reflexology every other day, the tear duct was cleared in less than a week.

One of our regular clients had her seven year-old grandson, Sammy, visiting her for the week. When he came down the stairs for breakfast, he was limping. His ankle was turned and he could not straighten it. It hurt when he put his weight on it. Of course, our client thought of Reflexology. She gave us a phone call and came by the office. I was with a client, so I only stepped out of the treatment room for a minute or two. I gave Sammy's foot and ankle a very mini "working" and his ankle was corrected immediately. On leaving the offfice, he said, "Gradma, that lady has magic fingers!" This client has suggested that we name this book "Magic Fingers."

# XIV. SCOLIOSIS

Definition: Scoliosis is a lateral deviation in a normally straight vertical line of the spine.

A four year-old boy with Scoliosis was brought to our office by his mother. This was our first case and we knew Reflexology could do no harm but we didn't know how much good it could do, either. He complained of his legs' aching and he was tired constantly. He couldn't keep up with any of his friends when doing physical activities. His mom brought him to our office for Reflexology therapy once a week. We didn't feel that once a week was going to give us the results we were striving for. We looked up Scoliosis in our professional textbooks in order to find what the medical profession was doing as treatment for Scoliosis. We found out that they recommended using braces less often and concentrating on improving the muscles to help support the spine. Muscle tonement! That is one of the areas in which Reflexology treats best, so working for the purpose of muscle tonement was the turning point! We showed Mike's mom where and how to work the most important reflexes on his feet. She did this briefly each night. Mike was improving, sleeping better and had fewer leg pains. His progress was checked by his chiropractor with x-rays. Reflexology had stopped the curvature from increasing and the x-rays showed a quarter of an inch improvement in the curvature of the spine. His mother took several classes and became a Certified Reflexologist. Today she not only does Reflexology for her son, but Reflexology has become her profession. At this writing Mike is now ten years old and shows almost no signs of Scoliosis. Our conclusion for treatment was that we should concentrate on the reflexes for the adrenals, all glands and the spine.

When we performed Reflexology to clients with Scoliosis, we found the following reflexes to be the most helpful: *whole spine, adrenals, all glands, chest/lung, shoulder, and the fifth zone.*

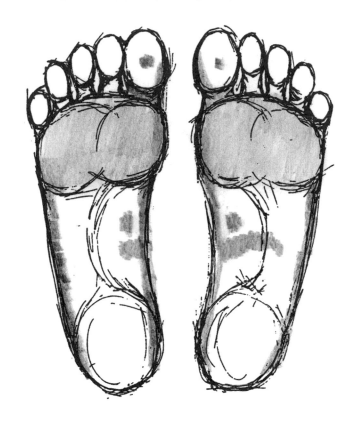

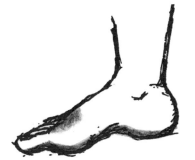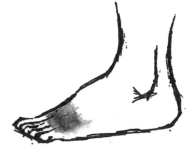

Page 60

# XV. CYSTIC FIBROSIS

Definition: Cystic fibrosis is a disorder associated with widespread dysfunction of exocrine glands, with the accumulation of excessive mucus and abnormal secretion of sweat and saliva.

Chrissy was twelve years old when her mother brought her to our office for Reflexology therapy. Her mother explained that the family was moving to Tennessee within the month and that the nearest hospital would be quite a distance from their new home. Chrissy had been receiving medical therapy twice a week to help her with her breathing and expectoration. Chrissy's treatments at the new hospital would not be as often, because of the distance and difficult transportation. Chrissy's mother wanted to learn how to do Reflexology in order to help her daughter between her medical treatments. Chrissy told us that her doctor showed her how to massage her "mucus valve" (Ileocecal valve area). We did some research on cystic fibrosis in order to know what the treatment, patient care and effects were concerning the disease. We read that some doctors were administering either hormones, enzymes, or animal pancreas as treatment. This helped us to better understand the disease and the areas on which to concentrate with our Reflexology treatments. Chrissy's breathing improved greatly with only three Reflexology sessions. Her mother took private classes in Reflexology at our office. After two weeks of twice a week Reflexology treatments, Chrissy's mother stated, "For the first time since I can remember, my daughter slept through the entire night without waking up, coughing and expectorating. I even got up to check on her to be sure she was all right."

Reflexology did help Chrissy with her breathing. Also, she had better elimination. One day, about a week before their move Chrissy came to the office for her usual appointment carrying a milk shake. I was shocked! "Milk can cause mucus" I told her mother. Her mother told me Chrissy received ice cream at the hospital after each of her breathing therapy treatments. Her mother did research on mucus forming foods and changed many of their eating habits. We received a card after their move, thanking us for our help and for showing them how to maintain better health with Reflexology.

When we did Reflexololgy to clients with cystic fibrosis, we found the following reflexes to be the most helpful: *diaphragm, lung/breast, ileocecal valve, adrenal and all glands.*

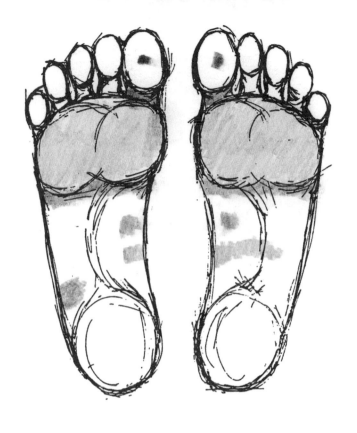

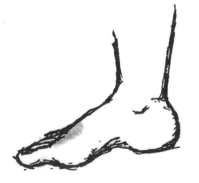 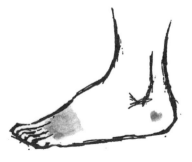

# XVI.  ALAGILLE SYNDROME

Definition: Alagille Syndrome is  genetic condition characterized by jaundice and erratic liver function, abnormalities in the cardiovascular system, the spinal column, the eyes, and the kidneys. The patient suffers with itching, fat deposits under the skin, loose stools, and stunted growth during early childhood. this disease can stabilize between ages 4 and 10 years with improvement of symptoms, but 40% of patients eventually need a liver transplant due to severity of organ function degeneration.

This case study is about a little girl born with Alagilles' Syndrome. When we met her she was just eight years old,  but her body was the size of an  average four or five year-old.  Lizzy's  liver was shutting down, causing less vitamin and mineral assimilation, more bile, more cholesterol, and more itch.  Poor little Lizzy  looked like one of the starving children in the third world.  Her stomach was extended and extremely hard to the touch. Her liver cholesterol and bile salts  made her itch so badly that she scratched herself continually.  Her grandmother had been a regular client of ours. Grandma began sharing her treatments with her granddaughter. They would receive a half hour Reflexology treatment each.  Lizzy was maintaining well.  Then she contracted a children's virus from her classmates, which her weakened immune system could not handle and as a result she became very ill.  We did not see her for weeks.  Her condition deteriorated until she was on the list for a liver transplant when one was available.  Grandma had to carry her when they came into our office again, as Lizzy was too weak to walk.  Her legs were extremely swollen, she couldn't put shoes on her puffy feet and the whites of her eyes were very yellow.  Poor Lizzy was almost listless. Beginning December 25, 1994 we worked on her three times a week for a full one-hour treatment. After the New Year we Lizzy daily for ten days.  Soon Lizzy was well enough to go back to school.  There was no more swelling in her lower limbs, her eyes were less yellow and her tummy was softer. Lizzy continued to receive one half-hour treatment twice a week. She maintained this schedule for more than a month. Even though Lizzy still needed a new liver, Reflexology therapy enabled Lizzy to be in the best physical condition that she had been in for a long time. One evening a call came to Lizzy's home telling her family there was a liver waiting for her in Chicago. The Lear jet arrived in Tampa to transport a liver transplant patient.

The medical personnel and crew were stunned to find a happy, dancing, singing child who did not seem near death.

Lizzy had the transplant the next day. Friends and family had donated twenty-nine pints of blood in Lizzy's name, but she only needed one pint during the surgery. She was in I.C.U. only 36 hours then she remained in the hospital for only twelve days. Whether or not Reflexology could have done more, we will never know. What we do know is that when Lizzy had extensive surgery, she was in the absolute best physical condition possible because of Reflexology. When she returned home she continued with her weekly Reflexology treatments to help with the healing process.

Paul and I wanted to give Lizzy a special gift. We arranged for Lizzy to go and see a lovely lady who makes dolls. Lizzy had a doll made to look just like her who she named Daisy. Since during Lizzy's recovery she was not able to play with other children, Daisy became her best friend. Lizzy even writes stories about Daisy and about all of the mischief they both can get into.

Lizzy is doing remarkably well. All of Lizzy's doctors are pleased with her progress and so are we. We realize that many Reflexologists would be afraid to do Reflexology on someone after a liver transplant. Please remember that Reflexology aids the body to 'normalize' and does nothing to harm the body, but rather can assist the body to stabilize itself. Reflexology has helped Lizzy to continue to be in the best physical condition.

Lizzy was granted a "Wish Come True" by the Suncoast Children's Dream Fund. She and her family went to Arizona to see the place where Lizzy was born, ride a horse, and be a cowgirl. At the time of this writing, it has been two years since Lizzy's liver transplant and all is well with her.

Lizzy says, "Everyone says I got better faster than most kids with a liver transplant. My whole church, friends, my school, my relatives, and people I don't even know rejoiced that I got well so fast. Lots of people prayed and called it a miracle. I know it was, too."

When we did Reflexology for Alagilles Syndrome , we found the following reflexes to be the most helpful: *liver, spleen, intestines, all glands, especially the pituitary.*

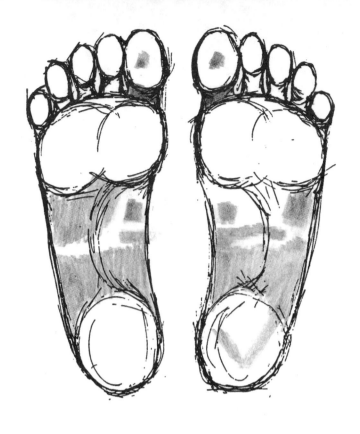

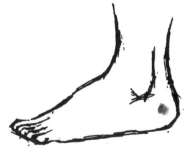

Page 67

# XVII. PREGNANCY

Definition: Being with child; having a developing embryo or fetus within the uterus.

Most of our pregnant clients are without specific problems. They receive regular treatments before and after their pregnancy. Reflexology can help pregnant women with their back discomfort, swelling or edema, and help maintain good blood supply to them and the unborn child. The glandular system can go "out of sorts" and what better way to balance the total body than with Reflexology!

We worked on a lady who, in her eighth month, was still swimming twelve to fifteen laps a day. Swimming had always been her way to exercise. She continued to receive her Reflexology treatments through out her pregnancy. Sometimes she complained of the back ache; sometimes it was mood swings. However, she always felt better after her Reflexology treatments.

I recall working the feet of a womcn whom I did not know was pregnant. Allison was extremely healthy, and showed no discomfort anywhere in her feet. I worked the reflex for the uterus and it was extremely sensitive. Allison was a student of Reflexology and just smiled. Then she told me that she had just come from her doctor's office and that she was a few weeks pregnant. The reflexes already showed the changes happening in her body. I knew about her pregnancy before the father did.

(1). Wendy was told by her doctor that her blood test showed her sugar level to be elevated. They were going to test again the following week, and if there was no improvement, medication would be necessary. Until now her pregnancy had been healthy. Wendy really didn't want to go on medication if there was an alternative. She received Reflexology treatments every day for one week. The new test results showed her blood-sugar-level to be within normal range. We showed Wendy's mother which reflex areas to work in order to maintain the results which she had gained. Her mother worked her feet every other day.

When Wendy went to the hospital to deliver her baby, her mother was with her administrating Reflexology therapy, in order to ease her discomfort and keep her relaxed. When Wendy felt the need to push the medical staff told Wendy not to push yet, because they felt it would be quite a while before her baby would be born. Everyone present was amazed when only ten minutes later she delivered a beautiful, healthy baby girl. Wendy and her mom swear that Reflexology kept her calm and relaxed throughout her delivery.

I would like to add that Wendy's mom was the person that introduced me to Reflexology by giving me my first book on Reflexology. I must thank her for introducing me to one of the loves of my life, Reflexology!

(2). June was a school teacher who was pregnant with her second child. Her doctors were very concerned because she had become very toxic. Her legs and feet were blown up like balloons. She wasn't scheduled to have a Caesarean delivery for another five weeks. Everyone was concerned for the health and well being of the baby. The doctors felt it could be dangerous if the baby was to be taken so early. June came to the office for one treatment and left with her shoes falling off; the swelling in her feet was gone. June went back to her doctor and asked, "Why didn't you recommended Reflexology for toxemia?" He stated, "Reflexology is unorthodox and I couldn't recommend it." However, he did tell her to keep doing whatever she was doing. June came weekly for the next few weeks and had no further problems with toxemia. She had her Caesarean delivery as scheduled. Every year June invites us to give a lecture to her class. It is always a pleasure to introduce young people into an alternative method for good health.

(3). We "worked" our daughter, Suzette, when she was pregnant with her first child. She was working full time as a pedicurist and when she came home from work, her feet and ankles were always swollen. Suzette would receive a short treatment nightly. I had the pleasure to be with her during her labor. Her labor was quite long, from 11:00p.m. till 10:00 a.m. At one point the nurse was concerned that the stress was hazardous to the baby. I was new to Reflexology and new to the birthing experience (by my own daughter). I had been rubbing her back, neck and shoulders. I finally went to her feet instead of her head and began doing relaxing techniques. When I "worked" the spinal twist technique, the baby's monitor immediately showed the stress level of the baby calm. Next, the mother's monitor showed that she had become more calm. Naturally, you are not going to stop the delivery.

How about helping nature to normalize? The labor and delivery were without problems. After Suzette delivered our beautiful little girl, Chantal, the doctor laid the baby on Suzette's tummy for her first of many kisses. Then the nurse wrapped Chantal up and handed her to me. I did touch every toe and every finger "working" light Reflexology.

When Paul and I returned to the hospital later that afternoon, we found our new grand-daughter lying in the nursery crying. Paul put on a gown and went to her side and began singing to her. You should have seen the nurses faces when Chantal stopped crying and became calm. You see, each night when Suzette got her Reflexology treatment, Paul would play his guitar and sing. His voice must have soothed and calmed our sweet grand-daughter in

When we did Reflexology to clients who were pregnant, we found the following reflexes to be the most helpful: *uterus/ reproductive system, all glands, spine, and diaphragm.*

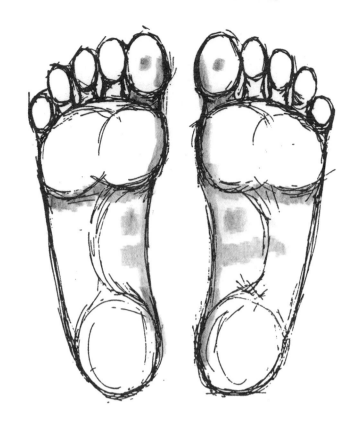

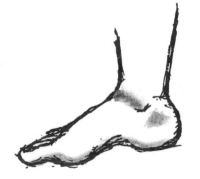 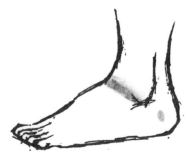

Page 42

# XVIII.  GYNECOLOGICAL  PROBLEMS

Gynecological problems may include:  endometriosis, menopause, or irregular menstrual cycles.

(1). Priscilla came to our office after being told by her doctor that she had endometriosis.  She had very painful menstrual cycles.  The doctor thought pregnancy would be difficult, if not impossible.  Priscilla began a series of Reflexology treatments.  We saw her twice a week for one month, awaiting her next menstrual cycle.  She was astonished at the lack of discomfort before and during her menstrual cycle.  Priscilla continued her Reflexology therapy once a week for another month.   She returned to the doctor for evaluation. The doctor felt that Priscilla's condition had improved greatly; therefore, pregnancy was no longer impossible.  I would love to state that she is now pregnant, but since Priscilla isn't married she is grateful to have pregnancy as part of her future.

(2). Leslie suffered from extreme headaches, nausea and pain during her menstrual cycles.  Every month she would lose work, because she would  have to spend a lot of time in bed.  Leslie received Reflexology twice a week for one month until her next menstrual cycle.  Even though her usual headache was gone she still had much discomfort, but she did not lose any work time.  We spaced her Reflexology treatments to once every week for the next month.  Leslie had no difficulty with her next menstrual cycle.  **Reflexology works!**

(3). A woman who was going through menopause complained of depression and dryness of the vaginal area. She had Reflexology therapy three times the first week and twice the next week. By the third week, she said her marital relations had greatly improved because there was no longer dryness of the vaginal area. Her depression had lessened and she was praising Reflexology as *her last resort.*


(4). Another woman in her thirties came into our offices because of chronic fatigue. She never wrote or mentioned that she hadn't had her menstrual cycle for two months. After the second Reflexology treatment she brought a beautiful eucalyptus arrangement to place over our office doorway. It was her way of thanking us, as her menstrual cycle had begun again.

When doing Reflexology for menstrual problems, you can't just work for one or two treatments. You usually need to work from one menstrual cycle to the next. By doing this, a maintenance program, which is right for the client, is established.

When we did Reflexology on clients with Gynecological Problems, we found the following reflexes to be the most helpful: *uterus, ovaries and fallopian tubes, pituitary and all glands, lumbar/sacral/ and the diaphragm.*

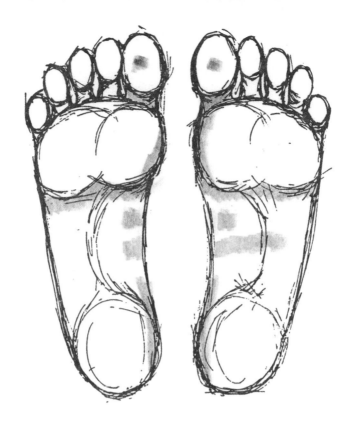

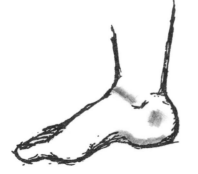 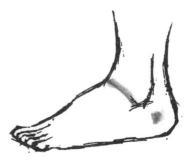

Page 75

# XIX.  GALLSTONES

Definition:  A gallstone is a stone-like mass, called a calculus, that forms in the gallbladder.  An excess of cholesterol in the bile appears to be of major importance in the formation of most gallstones.

(1).  Paul and I were at the local mall participating in a health fair when Matt came over to our booth, his body bent in half with both of his arms clutching his stomach.  Matt felt that he was having another gallbladder attack.  Matt told us that he and his wife were on vacation.  Matt's wife had seen us doing Reflexology to people at our booth while she had been shopping at the mall.  Matt said, " My wife rushed back to our  hotel and told me I had to go back to the mall with her.  I was familiar with Reflexology and was happy to get some relief."  Matt received a Reflexology treatment for one hour at our booth.  We suggested that he and his wife walk around the mall to be sure the pain would not return.  About one hour later they returned to our booth. Matt stated that he had to use the restroom twice to eliminate gas and have a bowel movement.  He had absolutely no more discomfort or pain.

(2).  Charlene came to our office suffering a great deal of discomfort. This was the same discomfort that she had previously experienced when she was diagnosed as having a gallbladder attack.  The reflexes in her feet showed that the colon reflexes were more sensitive than the gallbladder or liver reflexes.  After Charlene's Reflexology treatments she ·felt an urgent need to eliminate.  After the bowel movement, her pain was totally gone.

(3). We recently saw a new client who was considering gallbladder surgery. Wanda suffered pain after eating almost anything. When Wanda came back for her second Reflexology treatment, we asked how her digestion had been. Wanda paused for a moment, then said, "I can't remember any discomfort since my last Reflexology treatment."

(4). Karen was having gallbladder attacks nearly every night. She started receiving Reflexology every evening and within the first three treatments she had no more gallbladder attacks and her elimination had greatly improved. Karen received Reflexology once a week for several weeks and was pain free. She and her family moved to North Carolina and she ceased with her Reflexology treatments. She maintained good health for more than a month in North Carolina, then the attacks returned. The attacks were stronger and harder than previously. She ended up in the emergency room and was told that surgery was necessary. She returned home and made plans for her two little boys to be cared for. Karen had her gallbladder surgically removed. Even to this day, Karen feels that if she could have continued with her Reflexology treatments, it would not have been necessary to have her gallbladder surgically removed.

When we did Reflexology to clients with gallbladder problems, we found the following reflexes to be the most helpful:    *liver, gallbladder, thyroid, and the large intestines.*

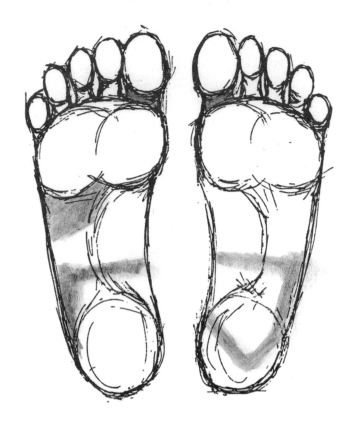

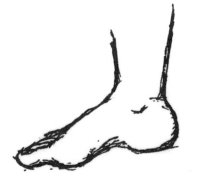

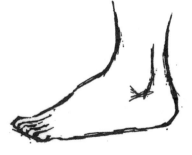

Page 78

# XX. STRESS

Definition: The biological reaction to any adverse stimulus, physical, mental, or emotional, internal or external, that tends to disturb the homeostasis of an organism.

(1). Stress made it impossible for Dale to sleep soundly. Dale had been in an explosion several years before coming to our office. He was in his mid-twenties when he was injured by a dynamite explosion, which threw him twenty feet into the air. He lost his left arm from the elbow down and his right hand had only a thumb and the stump of one finger. His right leg had been amputated and the explosion had left him blind. His face and chest had been reconstructed and he wore two hearing aids. His Reflexology treatment consisted of working whatever remained of his hands, feet, or extremities. Dale had not slept through the night since his accident. His nerves were a wreck. Dale was visiting his sister and she treated him to *one* Reflexology treatment. He didn't enjoy his treatment very much. There wasn't one area on his hands, foot, and stump that wasn't sensitive. About an hour after his treatment, his sister called our office. She said, " When we got home, Dale asked me to fix him a drink, as he lay down on the couch. When I returned with the drink, he had already fallen asleep and he is snoring! " The next day she called to say that Dale never woke up until the following morning. He had slept from four p.m. until six a.m. *Stress Relief!*

(2). A stressful job with too many long hours, burning the candle at both ends, and your body breaks down in some manner. Ellie was only thirty five years old and a manic depressant. A brilliant young women under medical and mental health care, and on many prescribed medications. Ellie actually slept through most of her first Reflexology treatment. She had tremors so badly that my chair was vibrating. She couldn't keep her arms on the arms of the reclining chair. Her arms would thrash and her legs and feet could not remain still. Ellie's father agreed to give Reflexology a try by giving her five treatments in two weeks as a gift. In just two one-hour Reflexology treatments her tremors were greatly improved. After her third treatment, Ellie no longer fell asleep and found the treatment to be quite sensitive. After her five sessions Ellie told me, "I know I'm getting well. I'm not sleeping my day away. I am afraid that this is too good to be true. I'm enjoying life again."


(3). Picture yourself as an executive in a fairly large corporation. You're told to fire one of the employees. It is your job to hire and fire, and he deserved to be fired; so, you tell him that he is fired. Later that day you're having lunch with several other employees when the disgruntled ex-employee, armed with a gun, approaches your table and opens fire. Some people are dead, some are badly wounded and you don't have a scratch on you. " Why me! Why am I not dead! I'm the one that fired him, you continue to say to yourself." Weeks go by and you can't sleep, you've become depressed and confused. This happened to Jay. Jay received psychological counseling in order to help him mentally adjust and to give him some relief from his nightmares. He wondered why he couldn't sleep and why his leg ached all the time? *Stress!* When Jay came for his first Reflexology therapy treatment at our office he had constant pain in his left leg and low back. The stress of the accident had taken its toll. On completion of his first three Reflexology treatments, Jay felt improvement with his leg pain. By the time he had received five Reflexology treatments he was able to get a good night's sleep again. This was a case where everything Jay had tried did not relieve the stress until he tried Reflexology. Jay came for seven consecutive treatments and then went on a maintenance plan of once a week. After several weeks he maintained with one Reflexololgy treatment a month. *Success at the last resort!*

When we did Reflexology on clients suffering from stress, we found the following reflexes to be the most helpful: *solar plexus, diaphragm, whole spine, adrenals, all glands, the fifth zone.*

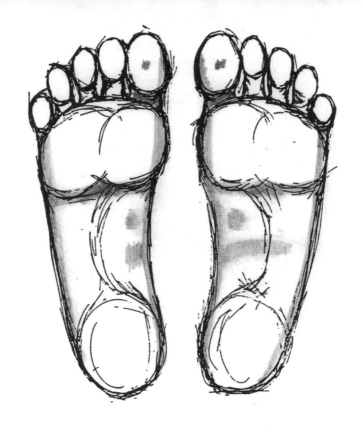

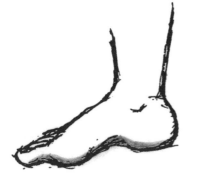
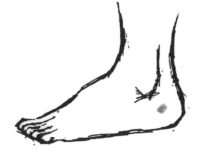

Page 82

# XXI. GOUT

Definition: Gout is an hereditary form of arthritis in which excessive quantities of uric acid appear in the blood and may be deposited in the joints. When this happens, there is swelling, inflammation, and extreme pain in the affected joint.

(1). Thomas had gout in his great toe. When he found out we were going to touch his toe, he nearly cried. He told us that when his bed sheet touched his toe the night before, the pain woke him from a sound sleep. "How are you going to touch that toe?" he questioned. "Very gently," I replied. I began by just placing both hands around the great toe, not even touching it, until some of the inflammation calmed in the toe. Then, very carefully and gently, I began working the area around the toe until I could actually work the great toe. During the middle of his first Reflexology session he had to use the restroom. After a Reflexology treatment of one hour he was able to put his shoe on and walk. He still had discomfort but not pain. He returned for two more treatments that week and hasn't suffered since.

(2). Gout doesn't always show up on the great toe. One client came to the office on crutches, unable to wear shoes. Gout had affected the entire top of his foot. Kile's foot was swollen from the ankle to the base of his toes. After his first Reflexology treatment, he was able to put his foot on the floor and did not have to rely on the crutches. The next day Kile returned for another treatment. After this treatment he left our office walking normally. By the third treatment, he was able to wear his work shoes.

(3). It was my understanding that gout didn't have to be in the great toe, but I thought it usually affected a lower joint. Milly came to our offices after being diagnosed by her doctor as having gout in her thumb. Who am I to question the diagnosis of a doctor? I began to do Reflexology on the affected area of her thumb prior to working her feet. Each time she received a Reflexology therapy session she had less pain and more mobility in the thumb. After four one-hour sessions, she had no more problems with her thumb.

When we did Reflexology on clients with gout, we found the following reflexes to be the most helpful: *kidneys and urinary system, and the reflex to the affected area.*

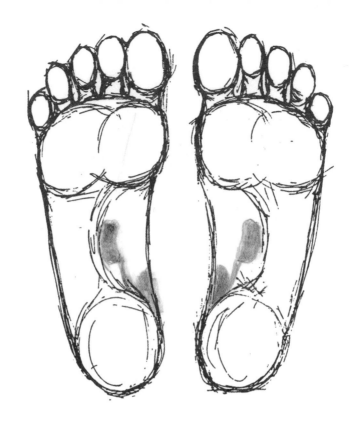

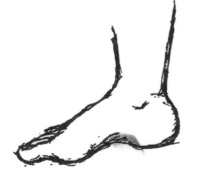
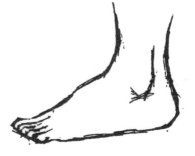

Page 85

# XXII. BELL'S PALSY

Definition: A paralysis of the muscles on one side of the face, usually caused by neuropathy of the facial nerve.

(1). Mable. Mable was in town for just one week. She had been diagnosed as having Bell's Palsy many years ago. The left side of her face had been affected. She was willing to come to our office for daily Reflexology treatments. While she was receiving her treatment we could actually see changes in her face. At first her left eye was extremely crossed; but, after the treatments continued, it was much more centered and appeared to be open wider than it previously had been. Also, she had experienced some drooping of her mouth, which diminished after several Reflexology treatments. We never received 100% restoration; however, a 70% improvement rate is quite a *success story* anytime!

(2). Carey. Carey was another lady with Bell's Palsy who received Reflexology treatments for overall improved good health. Her face drooped and her mouth was quite distorted when she talked. After three treatments she came to the office and declared, "I can turn my head!" We weren't aware that she couldn't turn her head. It had been three years since she was able to turn her neck to either side. We had concentrated on working the cervical reflexes to help the Bells Palsy, and in doing so we helped an unrelated problem, which we didn't know existed. After one month of Reflexology treatments twice a week, Carey's face had greatly improved and she no longer drooled out of the side of her mouth. Her Bell's Palsy was improved, and she could turn her head.

A few weeks later, she was being examined by her eye doctor, when he exclaimed, "Where did your cataract go?" *Success at the Last Resort!*

When we did Reflexology therapy on clients with Bell's Palsy we found the following reflexes to be the most helpful: *brain, cervicals, neck, side of neck, all toes and the diaphragm.*

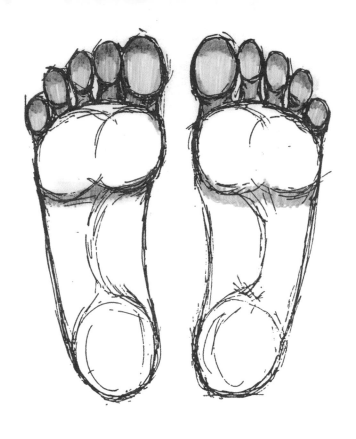

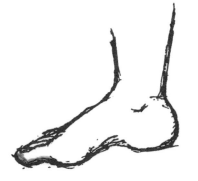
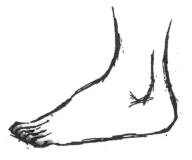

Page 88

# XXIII. COLON PROBLEMS

Reflexologists seem to get good results for clients who have problems with constipation, diarrhea and diverticulitis. There are many examples. Most of ours were not outstanding.

(1). Marcy. Marcy had experienced diarrhea for more than a week. Nothing she tried helped. Marcy's doctor put her on a diet of green apples and dry toast. She lived one hundred and fifty miles from our office, but she found someone to drive her to our office for a Reflexology treatment. The next day she phoned our office to announce she had experienced no further diarrhea, even with just one treatment. Reflexology helped her body to normalize.

Hemorrhoids are another colon problem that Reflexology has helped. No matter how bad the hemorrhoids are, some noticeable relief should be achieved with the first treatment. Stress can have an adverse effect on the color as well as that of the digestive system. If the hemorrhoids are extremely bad and painful it may take several treatments to achieve the desired results.

(2). Mack. Mack was a truck driver from Montreal, Canada who had driven a truck load of furniture to St. Petersburg, Florida. He was in great pain, caused by his hemorrhoids. He received two Reflexology therapy treatments in one day and was able to sit and drive his rig back to Montreal, Canada.

(3). Jane is in our chapter on Cancer. Once Jane was unable to eat solid foods, she began have problems with an irritable bowel. While receiving a Reflexology treatment, she mentioned that she was constipated and had not eliminated for three days. I explained the importance of the ileocecal valve reflex and how the actual organ worked. She would either have serious diarrhea or constipation. When wanted to tell me she had a problem, she would say the "The back door isn't working right." Her hospice team commented that Reflexology helped keep her pain down and to a minimum.

When we treated Reflexology clients with colon problems, we found the following reflexes to be the most helpful: *colon, liver/gallbladder, adrenal, diaphragm, chronic area up the inside of the leg, and ileocecal.*

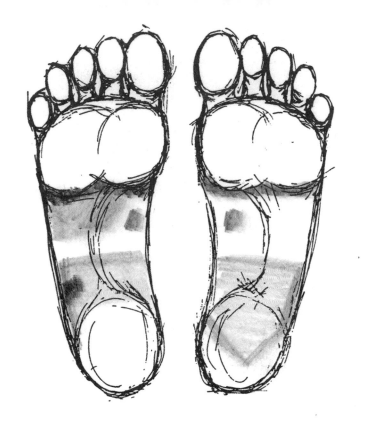

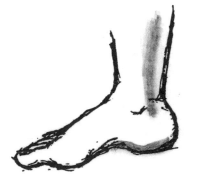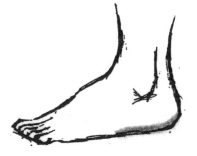

# XXIV. EARS

Some of the most common ear problems include: vertigo, tinnitus, dizziness, deafness, inflammation and plugged ears. Reflexology has helped many people with ear problems, a few are mentioned below.

(1). Connie. Connie came to our office complaining of her right ear feeling plugged or stopped up. She had been on vacation and traveled on planes many hours. Connie had experienced this feeling in her ear for two weeks. With each Reflexology treatment she felt improvement. After three treatments the abnormal feeling vanished.

(2). Jean. Jean said her right ear made her feel as though she was in an echo chamber. The reflexes to the neck ,cervicals and Eustachian tube were very sensitive, but the ear reflex was not. The condition disappeared after only two treatments of Reflexology therapy.

We have seen many clients experience improvement in their loss of hearing from Reflexology treatments. However, we've not been able to remove the need for existing hearing aids. We have known people who thought they needed hearing aids and after a few Reflexology sessions their hearing returned to normal. Many times the client doesn't come in for specific ear problems, but after treatment, he or she phones to say the dizziness is gone, or the ears are unplugged and their hearing has returned to normal.

(3). Marcia. Marcia received just one Reflexology treatment for her stiff neck.  Later that same day she phoned our office to say that the ringing in her ears was gone.  We didn't know she had ringing in her ears as she never mentioned it.

When we did Reflexology on people with ear problems, we found the following reflexes to be the most helpful: *ear, all toes, cervicals and neck.*

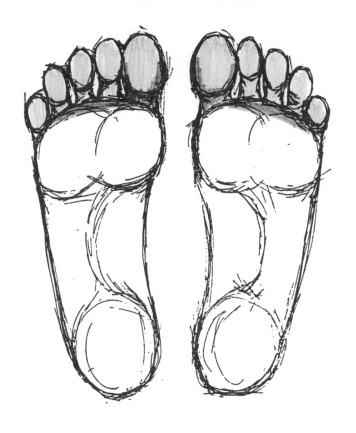

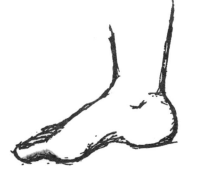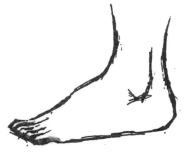

Page 94

# XXV. EYES

Reflexologists have thousands of stories about improved vision, disappearance of cataracts and easing of headaches around the eyes.

(1). Jake. We have seen two clients in the last five years who were scheduled to have eye surgery because a blood vessel in the back of the eye was dripping. Jake was a man in his late eighties. After six Reflexology treatments his doctor no longer found seepage from the eye; therefore, no surgery was needed.

(2). Homedi. She was about fifty-five years old and came to us after seeing an eye specialist. She wanted to see if Reflexology could improve her blood and nerve supply as well as help heal the vessel behind her eye, which was seeping. Homedi's neck reflexes were extremely sensitive and she was under a lot of stress at home. She received Reflexology therapy three times that week. When she returned to the eye specialist she was thrilled to learn she no longer had seepage behind the eye. Homedi is now a student of Reflexology.

(3). Sharon was forced to give up her drivers license, because she was declared legally blind. She heard about Reflexology and decided to see if there was any hope of improving her eyesight. We really couldn't promise success, because we'd never had a case like hers. Sharon received Reflexology three times a week for a month. Beginning with the first session we showed her how to do Reflexology on her own hands. We suggested that she work the eye/ear reflexes on her hands as often as possible. Sharon was determined and did the homework on her hands. She told us, " I work my hands every commercial, all evening long." Sharon is no longer legally blind and can drive a vehicle again. She still works on her hands every evening. We know Sharon helped us achieve the wonderful results we did with Reflexology. Sharon may wear thick lensed glasses, but she is no longer declared blind. Results at the *Last Resort!*

(3). Benson. Benson made an appointment at our office to see if Reflexology could help ease the pain in his left foot. He had pulled some muscles and was uncomfortable. After a series of five Reflexology treatments his foot was fine. Benson continued to get weekly Reflexololgy treatments. One day he came in for his treatment after he saw his opthalmologist had seen him. Benson told us that he saw his ophthalmologist every six months for the last three years because he had a small tumor behind his eye. If the tumor was to enlarge than surgery would be required. When the ophlalmologist could not find any sign of any growth behind his eye, he commented," I never saw this happen before, tumors don't just disappear". The doctor agreed that there are forms of natural health that are being used that have merit. Benson told him that the only thing he was doing was regular Reflexology treatments.

When we did Reflexology on people with eye problems, we found the following reflexes to be the most helpful: *eye, all toes, cervicals and neck.*

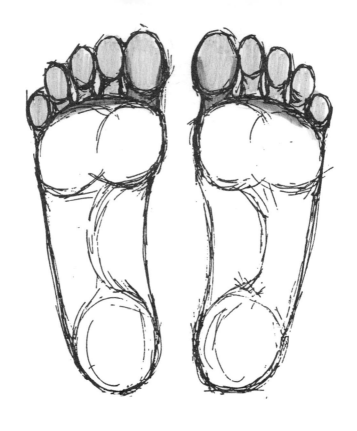

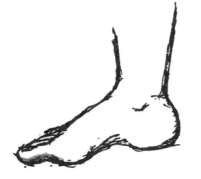
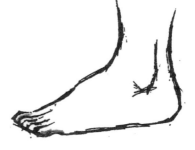

Page 97

# XXVI. PARKINSON'S

Definition: Parkinson's disease is a common disorder of the brain. It develops because of damage to the extrapyramidal nervous system; the part which controls movement, posture, balance, and walking. This damage results in the following primary symptoms: stiffness, tremors of resting muscles, slowing of voluntary movements and muscular weakness. We have only three cases.

(1). Lee. She came to our office in a wheel chair with her hands trembling uncontrollably. After one month of Reflexology treatments twice a week, Lee came to our office without her wheel chair. Lee felt Reflexology helped her control the shakes, and she felt stronger after each treatment. Lee walked fine until she had to cross a threshhold. She had difficulty getting through any doorway. It was as though her feet were glued to the floor and she couldn't move them. She had to be helped through the doorway. Lee continued with Reflexology treatments once a week for another month. She had regained much of her strength and had only a little trembling with her hands. She was able to walk through doorways on her own. Lee was such a refined lady that she was thankful that her dignity had been restored. She had hated the wheel chair. She has moved to another state, so we don't have information on her long-term results, but we do know that while she received Reflexology therapy she experienced a better quality lifestyle.

(2). Darlene. When she received Reflexology Darlene's arms and legs would thrash about uncontrollably. Paul had to forcefully hold her foot and continue to work the foot until the leg finally calmed down. She would stagger and bump into the walls in our hallway and had great difficulty lifting her feet. Darlene always needed assistance in getting from the car to our office, but <u>never</u> needed assistance going from our office to the car. The disease could not be reversed through Reflexology, but it helped her maintain a better quality of lifestyle for a few years. Darlene loved to dance and was able to dance only after her Reflexology treatments; so, she planned her treatments for the day her club was having their weekly dance. When she came in for her treatment she would tell us how many dances she had and how much fun she had. Darlene loved to do line dancing and the swing.

(3). John. John had difficulty with his speech, and suffered with great tremors. While doing Reflexology on his hands, his arms would thrash about and he could not control them. After a few minutes of Reflexology therapy on his hands his arms would calm and his tremors would almost disappear. He received Reflexology therapy twice a week for two months. John said, "Reflexology makes me feel stronger and more in control of my balance."

When we did Reflexology on clients with Parkinson's, we found the following reflexes to be the most helpful: *whole spine, brain, great toe, diaphragm, pituitary, all glands, all toes and the fifth zone*.

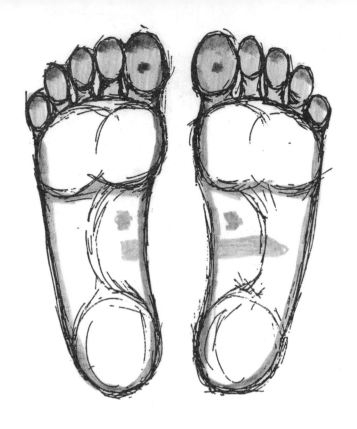

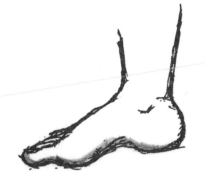 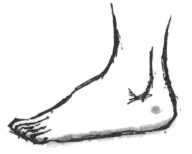

Page 100

# XXVII. URINARY PROBLEMS

Urinary problems may include: cystitis, incontinence, kidney stones, nephritis, or uremia.

During a Reflexology treatment, many times clients will excuse themselves because of the necessity to eliminate. After receiving treatments, it is not unusual for a client to say, "I no longer have to get up in the night to urinate. I can sleep through the night."

(1). Cindy: urinary tract infection. Cindy was only twelve years old. She had been having severe headaches and had seen several doctors. The doctors found no reason for her headaches except growing pains. As a Reflexologist, we could visually see the extreme puffiness around the bladder reflex area on her foot. The bladder reflex area was so tender to the touch, we could only caress the area gently for a few minutes. After the nerves calmed, we were able to give her a very gentle Reflexology treatment. Cindy had to urinate fifteen minutes into the treatment. She urinated three times in less than forty minutes. After the second trip to the bathroom, her headache was much better. By the end of Cindy's Reflexology treatment, her headache was completely gone. The next day her parents took Cindy back to the doctor and asked for a complete urinary test. The test showed a severe urinary tract infection. Why the headache? You've got me. Remember, people tell us their complaints to us, not the reasons for their complaints. Their feet will show the tender reflex areas that need attention. Cindy's feet indicated that the bladder reflex area was puffy and tender. Through Reflexology therapy we find the tender reflex areas, apply Reflexology techniques and the body normalizes. *Success!*

(2). Eva: kidney failure. Eva needed treatments three times a week order to be free from the kidney dialysis machine. Her condition was serious. When we first saw Eva she had no energy and was in a wheel chair. Her doctors told her that her kidneys were overflowing with protein. Eva's doctor wanted her to begin dialysis treatments within the week.

He told her that once she went on the dialysis machine, she might have two years to live. Eva received Reflexology therapy for a month. She and her doctor saw great improvement. The edema in her legs and feet would be completely gone after her Reflexology treatment. After a few days it would build back up again. We felt she needed at least two treatments a week. She and her husband simply could not afford it. Eva's husband was a carpenter, an eighty year old carpenter. My kitchen at home could use a carpenter! We purchased the materials and he did the work. After completing our kitchen, he retired. They couldn't believe that we didn't stop the treatments. We insisted that she continue with Reflexology twice a week for three years. Eva had improved to the point of being able to work in the yard. She even insisted on raking our new property which hadn't been raked in at least six years and we have twelve oak trees on the property. Eva worked in our yard every morning for a full week. This is the same women that came to us in a wheel chair. Eventually, they moved to another state in order to be near relatives. Six months ago (at this writing) she was put on dialysis. Her husband phoned us and said that she's not doing well. Reflexology did give her three years of extended living. I think that in itself is *Success!*

(2). Eva: kidney failure. Eva needed treatments three times a week order to be free from the kidney dialysis machine. Her condition was serious. When we first saw Eva she had no energy and was in a wheel chair. Her doctors told her that her kidneys were overflowing with protein. Eva's doctor wanted her to begin dialysis treatments within the week.

He told her that once she went on the dialysis machine, she might have two years to live. Eva received Reflexology therapy for a month. She and her doctor saw great improvement. The edema in her legs and feet would be completely gone after her Reflexology treatment. After a few days it would build back up again. We felt she needed at least two treatments a week. She and her husband simply could not afford it. Eva's husband was a carpenter, an eighty year old carpenter. My kitchen at home could use a carpenter! We purchased the materials and he did the work. After completing our kitchen, he retired. They couldn't believe that we didn't stop the treatments. We insisted that she continue with Reflexology twice a week for three years. Eva had improved to the point of being able to work in the yard. She even insisted on raking our new property which hadn't been raked in at least six years and we have twelve oak trees on the property. Eva worked in our yard every morning for a full week. This is the same women that came to us in a wheel chair. Eventually, they moved to another state in order to be near relatives. Six months ago (at this writing) she was put on dialysis. Her husband phoned us and said that she's not doing well. Reflexology did give her three years of extended living. I think that in itself is *Success!*

(3) Watts had been to the doctor several times due to an enlarged prostate. He had a lot of discomfort when eliminating and had to get up seven or eight times at night only to urinate a very small amount. He knew about Reflexology, but until his only option was surgery he had not tried a professional Reflexology treatment.

(3)    Watts had been to the doctor several times due to an enlarged prostate.  He had a lot of discomfort when eliminating and had to get up seven or eight times at night only to urinate a very small amount. He knew about Reflexology, but until his only option was surgery he had not tried a professional Reflexology treatment. Again, Reflexology was the Last Resort. After just one treatment he felt less discomfort when urinating. After the third treatment he came to the office praising Reflexology. He had gotten up only once during the night and had no discomfort at all. Watts received a series of Reflexology treatments, three times a week for two weeks. When he returned to his doctor for an examination, the doctor checked his prostrate three different times and was astounded that the prostrate that he had wanted to do surgery on was no longer enlarged.  Mike came to our office stating how he praises Reflexology and is telling everyone, he meant EVERYONE! He said that while he was in a public rest room he observed the man next to him did not have good output.  Then he mentioned he had experienced some prostate problems and that Reflexology therapy was the solution to his problems.


Living in St. Petersburg, Florida, is living in the retirement center of the United States.  We see many clients who complain about incontinence.  There have been many clients that have been helped with Reflexology treatments; however, we don't have any outstanding stories to share.  Most of them report that Reflexology has helped them to have better muscle tone for the sphincter muscle, and subsequently better control of the bladder.

When we give speeches at local meetings here, we always demonstrate to the people how they can help themselves by working the reflexes in their hands. We also encourage our clients to do the same, to help them get faster results. Dwight Byers calls it homework.

When we did Reflexology therapy to clients with bladder problems, we found the following reflexes to be the most helpful: *bladder, kidneys, ureters, adrenals, lower spine and <u>diaphragm</u> (if in pain)*.

(4). **Kidney stones**. Kidney stones are calculus (an abnormal mineral conretion in the body) in the kidney, which are composed of crystals precipitated from the urine on a matrix of organic matter.

Harold was hospitalized while waiting to pass one or more kidney stones. The stones were located where the kidney empties into the ureter. The doctors released him after three days; to go home and wait to pass the stones. Harold's wife was to examine the urine wearing rubber gloves to find the stones. The pain and discomfort when Harold urinated was almost unbearable. We went to his home and gave him a one-hour Reflexology treatment. During the treatment, we had to leave the room four times so Harold could use the hospital-type urinal. Harold had two one-hour Reflexology treatments the following day. He said the pain has lessened greatly and he wasn't eliminating as often. He also felt he had more control and that he could use the bathroom rather than the urinal. His wife examined the urine each time. Nothing. By the third day at home he had no discomfort at all. His wife told us, "Last night when I examined his urine there were little stone-shaped bubbles in it. When I touched them they dissolved." Harold went back to the hospital for tests to see where the stones were located. The tests could find no stones. The doctor asked Harold's wife if he had passed any stones. She told him about the bubbles she found. The doctor stated, "A stone is a stone is a stone. You will know it if you see one, I don't know what you saw, but it wasn't a stone." Whatever did happen, Harold didn't have to have surgery and Harold no longer had any discomfort.

When we did Reflexology on clients complaining of kidney stones, we found the following reflexes to be the most helpful: *kidneys, ureter tubes, diaphragm, parathyroid and bladder.*

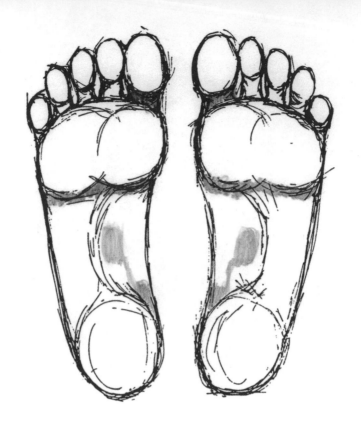

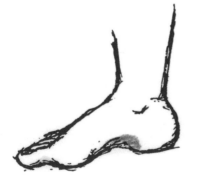
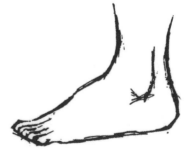

Page 108

# XXVIII. MULTIPLE SCLEROSIS (M.S.)

Definition: This is a chronic neurological disease. Symptoms can include weakness, lack of coordination, parasthesis, speech disturbances and visual disturbances. Stress due to trauma, infection, overexertion, and emotional upsets can aggravate the condition and even cause flare-up. We have three cases to share with you.

(1). Paulette. Paulette, a victim of Multiple Sclerosis, was a mother of three young children. When she came to our office, she was in a wheel chair. After Paulette received Reflexology treatments three times a week for two weeks she was able to walk with a cane. No more wheel chair! Her feet were extremely sensitive, and there were times when she would sing high notes rather than yell. One afternoon Paulette decided to play a joke on Paul. During her Reflexology treatment, she took her cane, screamed, then broke the cane in two. I ran into Paul's room to see what had happened. You should have seen Paul's face. When Paulette showed us that she had a collapsible cane we all had a good laugh. Earlier we mentioned that stress can cause exacerbation in Multiple Sclerosis patients. This was true with Paulette. The stress of raising three young children, not being able to work outside the home to help financially, plus her husband's disbelief in alternative health measures, made life very difficult for her. Paulette couldn't financially afford the necessary treatments, but neither could she physically afford to stop them. She had relapses when she didn't continue with regular Reflexology treatments. This was one of those cases where we charged for once a month and she received treatments once a week.

Paulette's family stress finally got the best of her and she stayed away for months. When we saw her again, she could no longer drive her car or stand on her own. Paulette was limited to her wheel chair! *Frustration!*

(2). Judy. Judy had suffered Multiple Sclerosis for many years. She received weekly Reflexology treatments at our offices for several years. When stress in her life caused exacerbation, we had to make house calls. Judy said, "Reflexology gives me more energy and strength. When I tried Massage, I felt like a wet noodle, but with Reflexology I feel invigorated." Judy recently moved, but she still receives Reflexology treatments on a weekly basis elsewhere.

(3). Jerry. Jerry is a self employed businessman. He has Multiple Sclerosis and the stress of the business world, as well as having teenagers to raise, does bring on exacerbations. Jerry had a major business deal in the making and could not afford to give in to his Multiple Sclerosis. He knew that with this added stress, he would end up in the hospital, if something didn't change. He was "a doubting Thomas," as far as Reflexology was concerned. Jerry came to the office for our money-back-guarantee and received five treatments the first week. Jerry didn't ask for his money back. He soon found that he no longer staggered into the walls and he had a lot more energy. Jerry received twenty Reflexology treatments in one month. We would suggest treatments every other day, but he was afraid to lose the energy and strength he had gained. Jerry's big business deal took him out of town for sometime, and when he returned he had even more stress with the added accounts. Because of this added stress and not receiving Reflexology to help counteract the stress, Jerry was hospitalized. I'm sure we will see him again soon.

I'm so pleased that this book wasn't finished, because Jerry called today and received the first of five new Reflexology treatments. He knows how much Reflexology has helped him in the past and is determined to gain his strength again. After his series of treatments, we asked him what he felt Reflexology does for him. He answered," I feel my gait, my balance and my equilibrium is better. I have better bladder control, my speech has improved and I have more strength. I have to credit my Reflexology therapy treatments to all of this. I know it has helped me and I am going to continue with my treatments."

(4) Marlene had been bed ridden for two years, because of M.S. She had had a colostomy and a permanent catheter. She phoned to see if Reflexology could give her some relief to the pain on her tail bone caused from inactivity. She was brought to the office and given a Reflexology treatment. The circulation in her feet and legs was not good. Marlene had poor muscle tone i in her calves, and her feet were swollen and very sensitive to touch. After her third session she was finding relief of pain on her tail bone. We encouraged to receive a series of Reflexology treatments twice a week for a month to help improve her muscle tone and to give her better strength. She began seeing results after the second week. Marlene was able to stay sitting upright in her wheelchair for six hours instead of lying in bed. Her feet and ankles were no longer swollen and she was indeed gaining strength. Marlene began taking natural health products, was strong enough to begin physical therapy, and continued with her Reflexology weekly treatment. Marlene can now stand on her own, and take three steps. She uses a motorized scooter (an Amigo) and is becoming independent instead of totally dependent on others. She and her wonderful husband can again go out to dinner. Marlene will tell you, " I credit Reflexology for making it possible for me to attain the ability to include other therapies. I thank Jesus every day for my continued progress." Results at "The Last Resort"

Here is an update on Marlene: Six months from her first Reflexology treatment, Marlene can walk from the van to the office with the aide of a walker. She isn't taking mini steps either, she is walking with strides the same as you and I would. She can dress herself, including her tie shoes and socks. She can even take several steps without the aid of the walker. She is about to regain her position as home maker. Paul and I are so please each time we see her, all we can do is smile.

When we did Reflexology on clients with Multiple Sclerosis, we found the following reflexes to be the most helpful: *whole spine, adrenals and all glands, brain, side of neck, the diaphragm and the fifth zone.*

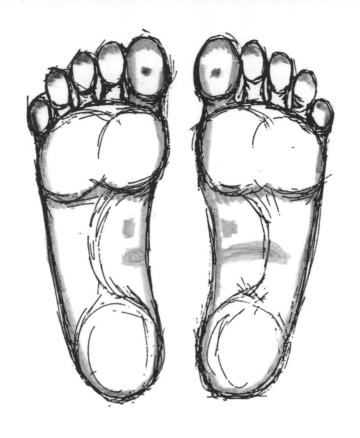

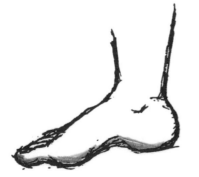 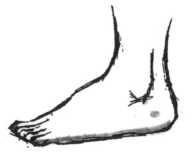

Page 113

# XXIX.  HUMAN IMMUNODEFICIENCY VIRUS, ( HIV )

Definition: Human Immunodeficiency Virus, is the virus that causes AIDS.  When someone becomes infected with Human Immunodeficiency Virus, the virus attacks that person's immune system. Only a specific blood test can tell if someone is infected with Human Immunodeficiency Virus. Only a doctor can diagnose AIDS.

We have worked on several people who  tested positive with the HIV virus. They all felt a  great improvement in their energy level after receiving Reflexology treatments. Since HIV affects the immune system, it is important that the client does not become weakened or overworked.   If their immune systems become weakened they need more Reflexology treatments closer together in order to compensate their bodies and have their immune systems restored or improved.  Reflexology can also help relieve stress and tension. If I tested positive with the HIV virus, I know I would have stress!

Paul and I know Reflexology can ease pain and discomfort. Most people who are seriously ill need to talk to someone. People try to remain strong for their family and friends. No one wants to see others crying and losing control. If you can remain calm during the Reflexology treatment, and allow the client to express any fears and discomfort, you will help him or her in two ways. Reflexology should help an individual rest more comfortably as well as to increase the energy level.  Most importantly, Reflexology therapy can aid the immune system to operate at its optimum level.

One of our H.I.V. positive clients receives Reflexology every three weeks. If he feels his coloring or energy is not normal for him, he calls to increase his sessions. After receiving a few more sessions in one week, he seems to have gained his energy and strength back. He lost a room-mate to AIDS, and doesn't expect to live a long life. He is living a better life with Reflexology than without Reflexology. That is *Success!*

When we did Reflexology on clients with HIV, we found the following reflexes to be the most helpful: *all glands, spleen, lymphatics and diaphragm.*

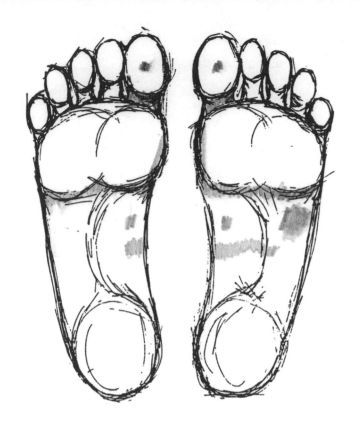

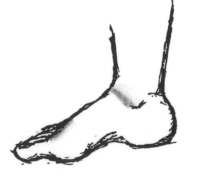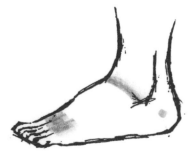

Page 116

# XXX.  CANCER

Definition: Cancer can be any malignant, cellular tumor. With this disease there is a transformation of normal body cells into malignant ones.

Most cancers, when diagnosed early enough, can be removed or treated.

We have had five different clients with lumps in their breasts. However, only one of those clients had cancerous lumps. The lumps on the non-cancerous clients all disappeared within five Reflexology treatments. It is truly amazing that you can actually feel a minute spot on the breast reflex, or on the top of the foot, in the same zone as the lump in the breast.

(1). Mona watched a small nodule appear on her hand as I was working a nodule on her foot. Both pea-like lumps were located in the same zone as the lump in her breast. It's amazing how our bodies react. By the third treatment the nodules had apparently disappeared, as no nodules could any longer be found on either the hands or feet. Her self examination showed no lump in the breast. She followed up with a visit to her doctor and was given a clean bill of health. Reflexology again produced balance in the body with excellent results.

A recent article stated that 85% of enlarged lymph nodes in the breast are just enlarged lymph nodes, not cancer.

(2). Lynn had a mastectomy a few years before receiving Reflexology. She had all of the lymph nodes under the arm removed. She was very concerned about some swollen lymph glands in her right groin area. Lynn was so afraid the cancer had spread. We suggested that she examine the lumps and determine what size they were. Were they the size of a grape, a quarter, or a small pea? This way we felt she could better determine if Reflexology was helping them diminish in size. She received Reflexology treatments twice a week for three weeks. The time came for her next checkup by the doctor. She lay on his examination table and asked him to examine the lumps in her groin. He tried to feel for the lumps. Lynn said, " Feel a little higher, a little lower, they have to be there!" She felt so stupid, for there were no lumps to examine. Because, she hadn't bothered to do the self-examination that we suggested. Her doctor gave her a clean bill of health.

(3). Beth had a radical mastectomy and removal of lymph nodes in her upper right arm. As a result of the surgery her right arm had ballooned and had become solid. Beth was having difficulty writing because her right hand was affected. She was concerned about keeping her job as a legal secretary. When we first saw her we were not sure how much Reflexology could help. This was a time to *experiment*. The arm had to have Reflexology techniques done on it, to try and soften the sold mass of tissue which had resulted. Her right hand and arm were three times the size of her other hand and arm. Beth's family saw improvement in the size of her arm after Reflexology treatments three times a week for two weeks. Her employer even commented about the difference in the size of her hand. The tissue had become softened and the arm had decreased in size. We felt lumps on the top of both feet in the breast reflex areas.

When Paul mentioned it to her, she told him that she had received breast implants after her mastectomy. Because of the many horror stories related to the side effects of silicone implants she subsequently had both implants removed. Beth continued to improve to the point that her right arm is only slightly larger than her left arm now. She continues to receive Reflexology therapy once a week.

(4). Jim didn't know he had cancer. He came to our office for Reflexology therapy to improve the circulation in his legs. While working on his right foot, we found a reddish/brown growth on the very center of the plantar of his foot. We questioned as to whether or not the growth hurt when touched or when he walked. He said it had been there quite some time, but it did not affect him. We didn't touch the growth, but did work all around it. We suggested that Jim see a doctor about the growth. Jim missed his next appointment and we didn't hear from him for weeks. He finally called to tell us that the evening of his treatment, while showering, the growth began bleeding profusely. He went to the emergency room because the bleeding wouldn't stop. After removing the growth his doctor told him that the best thing that could have happened was for the growth to open and bleed. The cancer had been contained and did not spread to the blood stream, which could have caused serious illness, possibly death.

(5). Rosa had advanced cancer when we first went to her home to give her a Reflexology treatment. She had cancer of the spine, and she suffered great discomfort. Rosa is a relative of a Reflexologist whom we know in Miami. We went to Rosa's home three times a week. It took over a hour to drive from our office to her home, so sometimes it was late in the evening before we could give Rosa a Reflexology treatment.

Each time Rosa received Reflexology her lower spine would relax and her headache would ease. Her husband said that every night after a treatment Rosa slept more comfortably. Her doctors had done all that they could and her prognoses was not good. With Reflexology, Rosa was able to sit up in her wheel-chair, instead of lying in bed. Rosa said, "After my Reflexology treatments I feel stronger, there is less pain, and the numbness leaves my legs. I sleep better after the treatments, and I need to talk to someone who is not too close to me. I appreciate Diane and Paul going the extra mile to help me; and, I appreciate Reflexology." We eventually showed her husband and her mother the most important reflex areas to help her to be more comfortable. They continue to do Reflexology nightly on Rosa and she is in less pain.

(6). Jane had been a client for several years. She first tried Reflexology for a neuroma on her foot, which no longer exists. She became a regular client receiving Reflexology treatments once a month for only a half-hour session.

In March of 1995 Jane was diagnosed with cancer on the floor of the mouth. She was given a 60% chance to live, if she would have surgery and Chemo- therapy. She said the doctor painted a very dismal picture for her future. He said he could operate and remove a large portion of her lower jaw, part of her tongue and the floor of her mouth. That would follow with Chemo, radiation and reconstruction. Her decision was to live the rest of her life, for however short it would be, as normally as possible. She refused all orthodox medical treatments. She did not want to change her diet or lifestyle. Since we had never had a client that was willing to receive <u>only</u> Reflexology therapy, we didn't know what Reflexology could do for her. We knew Reflexology could do no harm to her physically, and we hoped we could help ease any pain she was going to have. We asked her to receive treatments three times a week and to only pay for the first treatment each week. She agreed. The doctor gave her about six months to live. Her D-Day was August 16, 1995. The doctor agreed to give her pain medication if or when she needed it and would make himself available if she needed him. Jane takes an over-the-counter pain reliever at night to help her relax. She calls the cancer the crab. When we asked why she chose to call it the crab. She told us the word cancer in the Greek language means "the crab." She also mentioned the Zodiac astrological sign for Cancer is a crab. She could use the word "crab" easier than she could handle the word "cancer". First, the lower jaw started to swell and then a growth the size of a marble appeared on the outside of the cancer area. The growth grew and resembled a large boil with a core in the center. The core then began to seep and the growth continued to enlarge. The tissue around the growth began to thicken. When the growth became the size of a half dollar, it would erupt suddenly and bleed profusely for several minutes. The area around the growth became hard and discolored. The growth was a deep red color and the surrounding area was bruised looking in appearance. Each time she went to her doctor, he wanted to give her more pain pills. Jane told him she had no pain at all. He couldn't believe her. He went so far as to tell her that he could see her pain in her eyes and he wanted her to be honest with him. Jane swore to him that she had no pain. He was amazed. Jane was so pleased that she sat and figured out how much money she saved by not needing the Tylenol "threes." She had saved one thousand, two hundred twenty dollars and sixty-seven cents. Believe it or not, she gave us a check for that exact amount. She also pays for all of her treatments now, three times a week. This is a rare opportunity to see what Reflexology can do for cancer when someone is doing *nothing else to change their lifestyle*. It works!

Jane has been seeing her medical doctor every two weeks for the past two months. Last week her doctor told her that she wanted to remove the cancer growing on the outside of her face. The growth has reached about a three inches in diameter on the surface and up to six inches under the skin. The growth began bleeding profusely. One day at our office she removed the bandage so we could take a picture of the change in shape and size. Jane stood at the bathroom sink for at least four minutes with a steady stream of blood flowing. The bleeding would happen whenever the pressure would build. Sometimes it would bleed once a day and sometimes several times a day. The bleeding had lessened and she decided to take a shower. She told me later, " I was in a horror movie this morning. I was shampooing my hair in the shower and when I put my chin down and there was blood everywhere. The picture was grotesque. I had no choice but to stand there in the shower in a pool of my own blood until the bleeding stopped." It has now been more than a week since the last occurrence of bleeding. The bleeding is the reason the doctor wanted to remove the growth. Jane has decided that the surgery would be the beginning of her pain and the beginning of her hospital stay. She has refused surgery. Her doctor is not pleased but remains as her doctor.

Jane's crab is having a "junior". There is another growth attached to the original crab. The original crab does not bleed at all anymore. With each new growth pressure builds until the growth bleeds. I personally saw Jane fill one cup and part of a second cup with the fluid and blood when one of the growths erupted. In the period of time it took to remove the cup from the bathroom and take it to the kitchen the fluid had already jelled.

Jane saw a doctor of Radiology, and they discussed the possibility of treating the growth with radiation to attempt to stop the bleeding and hopefully shrink the size of the growth.

Jane agreed to the radiation and after receiving two series of radiation, the growth has disappeared. She still has the original cancer on the floor of the mouth. It has been a full year and six months since she was told she was terminal and would be suffering with pain. Jane has yet to have pain and she is still alive, we believe, due in part to the many Reflexology treatments she received. It works! It's beneficial! It produces positive results in many, many people.

At this writing it has been two years and three months since her diagnose of terminal cancer. Jane is indeed terminal. The tongue and mouth and very enlarged and tender. She can no longer eat even soft foods, but can still take in liquids. People that don't know her can not understand her speech, but her friends can. She still drives her car and has Reflexology treatments three times a week. The only pain pills she has taken up till not is liquid Tylenol. I know that it is just a matter of time and I will miss my friend Betty. I am thankful to God that I was able to help her with Reflexology and by being there for her.

When we did Reflexology on cancer clients we found the following reflexes to be most sensitive and, therefore, most helpful: *all glands, spleen, lymphatic, corresponding areas, brain (for increased endorphins), and diaphragm*.

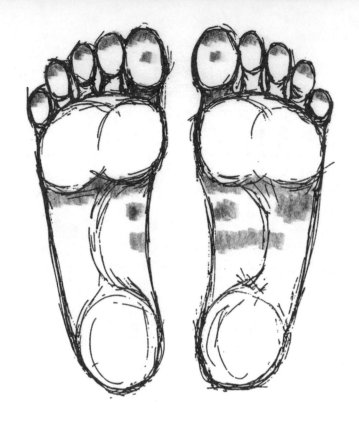

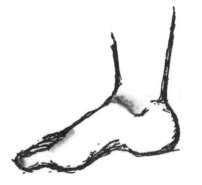 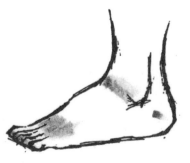

Page 124

# XXXI. TEMPOROMANDIBULAR JOINT SYNDROME, T.M.J.

Definition: A dysfunction of the temporomandibular joint, marked by a clicking or grinding sensation in the joint and often by pain in or about the ears, tiredness, soreness, and stiffness of the jaw muscles.

(1). I can personally testify to the results Reflexology can have on T.M.J and the jaw. Not only did I have severe T.M.J., but I had my lower jaw broken and extended. My doctors were amazed at the lack of pain and quick recovery I had experienced. Each time Paul gave me a Reflexology treatment to help relieve the discomfort, I could feel the joints relax, my face calm and the pain ease. First, I felt warmth, then tingles. I had three major surgeries on my lower jaw in three months. I met a women who had the same surgery about the time I had my first surgery. She complained that she still had swelling and numbness. I had experienced swelling and numbness for only two weeks, not six months. Again, Reflexology improved the blood and nerve supply allowing rapid healing.

(2). Marcia was seventy years old when she had to wear braces on her teeth to help alleviate the pain caused by T.M.J. Her dentist felt she would have to wear braces for at least three years. Marcia felt she was too old to go through all the discomfort of wearing braces, but she was too young to stop eating. Each time her orthodontist adjusted the braces she suffered a great deal of discomfort. Marcia would have headaches, earaches and face pain. She decided to try Reflexology treatments to help relax her joints and to ease the discomfort. Each time she received a Reflexology treatment, she noticed a remarkable improvement when her face relaxed and the pain lessened.

(3). Barbara wore braces and surgically had her lower jaw decreased. Barb's surgery was the exact opposite of mine. It had been at least six months since her surgery and she still had numbness in the front of her chin. Barbara is one of our winter visitors and when she came to Florida she arranged for several Reflexology treatments at our office. While getting her first Reflexology treatment she felt tingles and wiggly sensations in her chin and jaw area. Barbara commented, " I feel like little electrical currents or sparks are going through my face. " She had Reflexology four times in one week before returning to New York. Barb was amazed that in just one week her chin had regained 80% of feeling. Her entire jaw felt much more relaxed and she could open her mouth wider. I do love *success* stories!

When we did Reflexology to clients with T.M.J., we found the following reflexes to be the most helpful: *side of the neck, cervicals, base of the great toe, all toes and eye/ear reflexes*

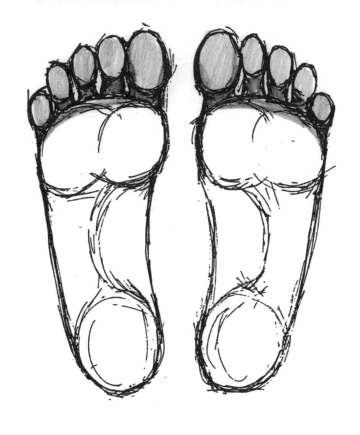

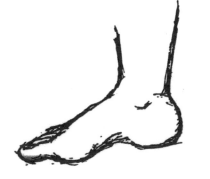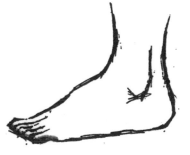

Page 127

# XXXII. KNEES

(1). I remember a gentleman who was very upset that he had his appointment with the <u>little</u> lady (Diane) and not <u>the man</u> (Paul). He even refused to write down any maladies, ailments, problems or reasons for wanting a Reflexology treatment on his questionnaire. He wouldn't even speak to me during the first half of the treatment. When I had finished his right foot and began on the left, he kept wiggling his toes on the right foot. I asked if he was waving at me. Wiggle, wiggle, wiggle,-he kept on moving those toes. Then he gave me a broad smile. He said that he hadn't been able to move any of his toes since he had his knees replaced six months earlier. Needless to say, he was no longer upset with the little lady giving him his treatment. He had two Reflexology treatments twice a week for three weeks. He was very happy to be able to go dancing again. Success in spite of himself!

(2). A medical student who was studying to be an orthopedic surgeon, came to our office because he had knee pain. He didn't want surgery because he knew that it could cause nerve damage. (I'll bet he won't tell his future patients that.) He received two Reflexology treatments and was amazed at the relief. His girl friend was going to try to continue giving him treatments in the future.

(3). Ellie has had two hip replacements, a shoulder replacement, and was in need of having a second shoulder replacement. Ellie's hips didn't hurt, one shoulder was fine and upon completion of the second shoulder replacement she should no longer be in pain. However, she is in continual pain. What is causing this pain? Ellie's knees! They will be the final chapter in her many surgeries. How does Ellie keep the pain level down? Her answer is Reflexology. We know we can't replace the cartilage and worn-out bone matter, but Reflexology can ease the pain and discomfort until the doctors repair the damage in her knees.

We have seen many older clients with complaints about the knees. Some have had knees drained, repaired, or even replaced. Reflexology can help ease their pain and discomfort. Even if surgery is necessary, we can improve the blood and nerve supply to the area. This should aid in their recovery.

When we did Reflexology on clients with knee pain, we found the following reflexes to be the most helpful: *hip/knee, hip/sciatic, lower spine, and the outer fifth zone.*

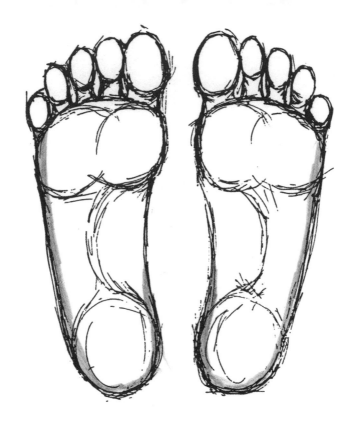

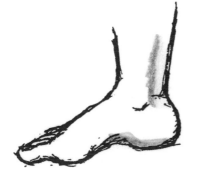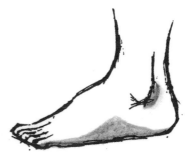

Page 130

# XXXIII. NERVE DAMAGE-1. Gullain-Barre' Syndrome
## 2. Neuropathy

**(1). Gullain-Barre' Syndrome** is a relatively rare disease affecting the peripheral nervous system, especially the spinal nerves, and sometimes the cranial nerves.

Alice was vacationing in Florida and came to our office for a Reflexology treatment. Her husband is a medical doctor. She said she had Gullain-Barre' Syndrome and wanted to know if Reflexology could help. "We don't know, but it can't do any harm", I said. The cranial nerves were affected and one side of her face appeared similar to that of someone suffering with Bells Palsy. She had suffered with this disease for more than twelve years. Her doctors felt that whatever damage remained was permanent. Alice received only four Reflexology treatments before she could see the difference in her mouth and left eye-lid. Her face even felt different to the touch. Alice swore that she would continue with Reflexology when she returned home. When I researched this disease, I found only one book which stated that nerves can restore or form a bypass if stimulated to do so. We feel Reflexology has that ability by improving blood and nerve supply to the damaged area.

**(2). Neuropathy** is a general term denoting functional disturbances and pathologic changes in the peripheral nervous system.

Mildred was diagnosed by her doctors as having Neuropathy of her lower legs and her feet. Her doctor told her that it was not caused by her diabetes, but from an auto accident in which she was a victim. Mildred's mother had taken a Reflexology class from Eunice Ingham years earlier, and the entire family used some Reflexology. However, this was the time for a professional Reflexologist and not just family play. Mildred was amazed at her results after just one Reflexology treatment. She returned four more times for a total of five treatments. Her Neuropathy had greatly improved and her pain was now only slight. Mildred is able to wear regular shoes for the first time in four years. She continues with regular Reflexology therapy at our office once a month, and receives weekly treatments from family members.

(3). Reflexology does not always work to the degree that we expect or hope. We extensively tried to help one eighty year old women through Reflexology treatments. Ellie received Reflexology therapy twice a week for two months. She had suffered from Neuropathy for ten years and the damage was extensive. When Reflexology wasn't able to give her the level of comfort we had all desired, we offered to return all of her money. Ellie wouldn't hear of it. She felt Reflexology had helped to improve her blood circulation and had helped her to sleep more comfortably. Two years later, she invited us to give a speech here locally for a social group at her condominium. Ellie told the group, "Reflexology couldn't help my Neuropathy, but it helped me in other ways. The thing I like best about Paul and Diane is the fact that they tried and were even willing to refund my money. I paid them for their hard work and loving efforts."

(4). We have been seeing Peggy since 1985. She had a chemical accident while at work. Lye was poured over her lower extremities. The accident resulted in major skin grafting and a lot of nerve damage from her knees down. Her insurance paid for any therapy that could give her relief from pain. Reflexology was the only therapy that could keep her mobile and in as little discomfort as possible. Her legs, where the skin was grafted, have now been restored to their normal color and the texture has improved greatly. Peggy usually receives Reflexology once a week. She stays active, always doing for others, and caring for the elderly. She is a super nice lady that found results at *the last resort.*

When we did Reflexology on clients with Gullain-Barre' Syndrome or Neuropathy, we found the areas most sensitive and most helpful to be: *the brain, great toe, spine and diaphragm.*

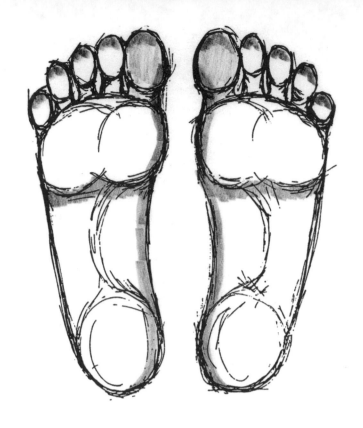

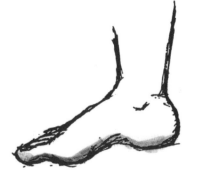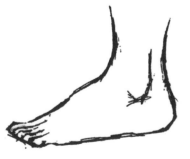

Page 134

# XXXIV. CONGESTIVE HEART FAILURE

Definition: This is a broad term denoting conditions that occur as a result of impaired pumping capability of the heart and is associated with abnormal retention of water and sodium.

This is about a gentleman whom we will call Dennis. Eleven months ago he was diagnosed and hospitalized with congestive heart failure. He was hospitalized for two weeks, at a total cost of $60,000. The results were that there was extensive damage to the back of his heart.

Late one evening, Dennis' wife phoned to see if we were home and willing to give him a treatment. His symptoms were similar to those of eleven months ago. Dennis refused to go to the emergency room. He wanted to wait until morning and contact his doctor. His wife brought him to our office. Dennis was gasping for air and with each breath you could hear the fluid gurgling inside his body. His coloring was gray; he could hardly speak. Paul began working Dennis's feet, while I was in another room talking to his wife. She said his condition had been deteriorating for two weeks. She felt that she would have to take him to the hospital before the night was over. When she and I finished talking, we joined the men in the treatment room. Dennis' condition hadn't improved so far. I decided to work his hands while Paul continued to work his feet. Dennis felt his chest calming and said that he knew we were helping. We continued to do Reflexology on both his hands and feet for an hour before his rapid, shallow breathing began easing. Paul and I worked on Dennis for one hour and forty-five minutes non-stop. His coloring had improved, his breathing was more even, his speech was less labored and the rattling fluid sound inside his chest had lessened

Page 135

somewhat. Dennis had to use the rest room before leaving. When he had finished, he commented, "I thought I would never stop, I kept going and going. I felt like the pink rabbit whose batteries keep going and going." He went home feeling a great measure of relief. He spent most of the evening sleeping in a reclining chair while his wife slept on the couch.

When he awoke early the next morning, he felt well enough to lie down in his bed. Dennis slept in his bed with his head elevated for several hours. Later that same day, he came to the office for another Reflexology treatment. Before his treatment he said, "I feel 80% better than I did yesterday." He was a different man! He felt much better than he had in the past two weeks. Dennis says, "I don't have a doubt in my mind, that I was on my way to another heart attack. Thanks to Reflexology I avoided it." After his second Reflexology treatment, he felt 90% better. Today Dennis feels 100%! It has been nine months since his severe attack. Dennis continues to receive Reflexology therapy twice a month. *Success!*

When we did Reflexology on clients with congestive heart failure, we found the following reflexes to be the most helpful: *the diaphragm, heart, lung, spine, urinary system and lymphatics system.*

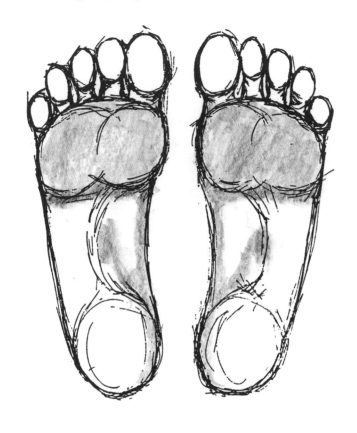

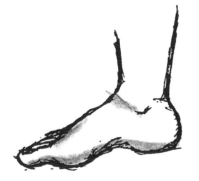 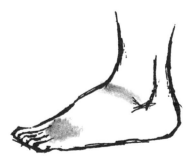

Page 137

# XXXV. NEUROMA

Definition: A neuroma is a tumor or new growth that is largely made up of nerve cells and nerve fibers. The following cases all had neuromas on their feet between the metatarsals.

(1). Joan is a teacher who suffered from a neuroma on her left foot. She was unable to stand for any length of time without sharp pain. Joan had read an article about Reflexology and thought she might like to try it since the neuroma was on her foot and Reflexololgy therapy is performed on the feet. There was a large mass between the third and fourth metatarsal bones. To the best of our knowledge, Reflexology therapy should break up the congested area and allow the body to reabsorb the built-up tissue and help the body to normalize. After each treatment, Joan felt less discomfort while standing on her left foot. Joan received five consecutive Reflexology treatments and no longer had any problems with the neuroma. *Success.*

(2). George had suffered from neuromas before. He had already been given the prescribed amount of injections of cortisone and gotten some relief. His relief only lasted three months and the discomfort returned. This time George decided to try Reflexology before going through the injections again. After only three Reflexology treatments George saw results. George has no more discomfort from his neuromas. Reflexology not only relieved the discomfort caused from the neuromas, but George saw a great difference in his calves. His calves previously felt tight and solid. He had difficulty walking without discomfort. By improving the blood and nerve supply to the body Reflexology therapy was a *success.*

We're not stating that all neuromas can be dissolved by Reflexology therapy, but we have not come across one that hasn't been helped. We know there are some that must be surgically removed. However, we are grateful that all of our clients with neuromas have not had to undergo surgery, and achieved results with Reflexology instead.

When we did Reflexology to clients with a neuroma, we found the following reflexes to be the most helpful: *area of the neuroma, lymphatic, pituitary and all glands.*

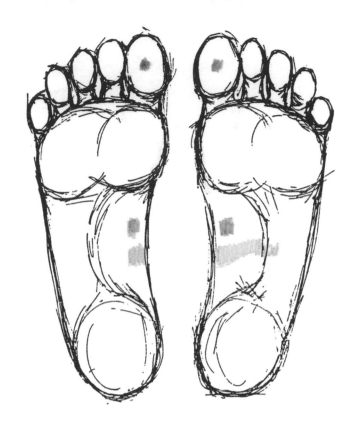

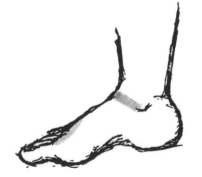 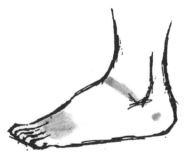

Page 140

Glossary:

Better Health with Reflexology, by Dwight Byers
Anotomy and Reflexology Helper Areas Study Guide, by Dwight Byers
Structure and Function in Man, by Sanders
Atlas of Anotomy, by Weston M.D.
Encyclopedia and Dictionary of Medicine, Nursing,
     and Allied Health, by Miller and Keane

A special thank you to Elizabeth Stevens for her editing advice.